AILING IN PLACE

AILING
IN PLACE

Environmental Inequities and

Health Disparities

in Appalachia

Michele Morrone

OHIO UNIVERSITY PRESS • ATHENS

Ohio University Press, Athens, Ohio 45701
ohioswallow.com
© 2020 by Ohio University Press
All rights reserved

To obtain permission to quote, reprint, or otherwise reproduce or distribute material
from Ohio University Press publications, please contact our rights and permissions
department at (740) 593-1154 or (740) 593-4536 (fax).

Printed in the United States of America
Ohio University Press books are printed on acid-free paper ∞ ™

29 28 27 26 25 24 23 22 21 20 19   5 4 3 2 1

Hardcover ISBN: 978-0-8214-2420-9
Electronic ISBN: 978-0-8214-4077-3

LCCN: 2019058666

Library of Congress Cataloging-in-Publication Data available upon request.

Contents

Preface   vii

Introduction to Appalachian Place and Health   1

CHAPTER 1   Foundations of Environmental Health   19

CHAPTER 2   A Place for the Built Environment and Health   39

CHAPTER 3   A Place for Water   58

CHAPTER 4   A Place for Food   75

CHAPTER 5   A Place for Pollution   92

CHAPTER 6   A Place for Resource Extraction   107

CHAPTER 7   A Place for Disasters   126

Epilogue
    Ailing in Place   142

Appendix 1
    Summary of the Environmental Health Profession
    in Appalachian States   151

Appendix 2
    Summary of State Agency Involvement in Select
    Environmental Health Programs   153

Discussion Questions   155

Notes   161

Resources   183

Suggested Further Reading   187

Index   189

Preface

I was not born in Appalachia, but I have a strong connection to the region. My family has roots in western Pennsylvania as part of the influx of immigrants from Italy and Eastern Europe. My maternal great-grandmother came to America from Czechoslovakia through an arranged marriage, settling in Johnstown in the early 1900s. Her daughter married my grandfather, who I never met because he died from silicosis when my mother was a teenager. My paternal grandfather immigrated from Italy as a child with his mother and settled in western Pennsylvania. He was a coal miner until he broke his leg, then he moved to Altoona and began a long career with the railroad as a car inspector. My father left Altoona for the same reason people leave Appalachia today: the economy was in decline and there was a promise of work near Philadelphia. I could never have imagined that my professional road would lead me back to these Appalachian roots, but I am grateful it did.

This book is the result of more than twenty-five years of work with and research about environmental conditions in Appalachia. My first job as an environmental professional was in 1992 as a planner assisting communities with sewage problems. One of my first projects was in southeastern Ohio in one of the thirty-two designated Appalachian counties in the state. I had been in this part of the state before, but this experience opened my eyes to the substandard environmental conditions in the area. It was also a defining moment because it pointed me in the direction of exploring how and why environmental conditions are different in Appalachia than other parts of the country. As I moved from environmental practitioner to public health academician, my curiosity about differences in Appalachia grew, and a new question began gnawing at me. I wondered how distinctive environmental exposures in rural Appalachia could affect the health of people in these places.

My curiosity about Appalachia was piqued when public health professionals began to document the connection between where people live (place) and their health. This led me to ask questions of the people who live and the professionals who work here. The topics in this book emerged from this combination of exploring data and talking to people. As I started digging deeper into circumstances with each of the topics, I thought I might find evidence of inequitable environmental exposures in Appalachia, and in almost every case I did. Most of the stories in this book arose from interviews and surveys of both residents and environmental health professionals. Stories of exposure to unsafe drinking water, inadequate food supplies, unsanitary conditions from floods, and contamination from industrial accidents are unfolding in places throughout Appalachia. These stories help us understand the environmental health concerns of the region and may explain why health disparities exist.

Once I found enough information to suggest environmental exposure inequities, I questioned whether these inequities led to health disparities in Appalachia. Discussion among public health researchers and professionals about health disparities began almost simultaneously to those about place-based exposures. Researchers were documenting health disparities in Appalachia in terms of conditions such as diabetes and cancers, and they were specifically focusing on how behaviors contribute to these conditions. I saw a gap in this research because so little of it was examining possible environmental contributions to health disparities. Helping to fill this gap is the motivation for this project.

My main purpose with this book is to raise questions about and draw attention to the connection between inequitable environmental exposures and health in Appalachia. For some readers, there is probably little that is earth-shattering here, and the questions I explore have been answered. On the other hand, some who work in the field of environmental health will say that it is not possible to definitively link environmental quality with health disparities. What I attempt to do here is provide evidence through both data and stories to show that Appalachian people are ailing in the place in which they live and not all health conditions can be explained by individual behaviors. If we accept this is the case, then we must argue for resources and policies to address poor health that results from systemic environmental degradation rather than personal decisions to eat unhealthy foods, smoke cigarettes, or refrain from exercise.

I would like to acknowledge Lucy Diavolo, who edited and contributed to this work. She provided insight and perspective from the eyes of a young person who has seen some of the environmental health impacts in the region. Ted Bernard, a trusted colleague and amazing author, also provided fresh insight and perspective. His guidance led to significant revisions with an eye to making it appeal to a wider, nonacademic audience. In addition, I am grateful to the hundreds of environmental health professionals who live and work in the region for participating in interviews and surveys about their work. Finally, the people of Appalachia with whom I have had the opportunity to interview and interact for the last twenty-five years have inspired me to do what I can to raise questions about environmental inequities and health disparities.

I would be remiss not to comment on the current status of environmental science in the United States. When I started this book in 2014, it was a different time in America than when I am finishing it in 2019. Federal environmental and public health agencies had different priorities than they do now. Science was valued and access to data was paramount. The change in administrations after the 2016 election had important consequences for those of us working to protect public health. One of the consequences is that some of the documents and research reports I relied on in the initial draft of the book are no longer readily available. This is especially the case when it comes to records and publications from the US Environmental Protection Agency (EPA). On September 17, 2018, I typed "EPA climate change" into the Google search bar. The appropriate agency page read, "This page is being updated. Thank you for your interest in this topic. We are currently updating our website to reflect EPA's priorities under the leadership of President Trump and Administrator Pruitt." Leaving aside the fact that on September 17, 2018, Administrator Pruitt was no longer at the EPA, this is just one example among many illustrating that there is no longer access to decades of good science conducted by the EPA.

Introduction to Appalachian Place and Health

> The first [word that comes to mind] is just the geography,
> that it's a region that stretches from Maine down the eastern
> seaboard of the country, down all the way to the South. And
> beyond that, because it implies difficult traversing terrain, rural
> isolated communities, strong independent people who don't
> really want to be messed with, who are not necessarily happy
> to change, but have a very strong sense of self-identity—which,
> you know, conflicts with change. An area that had been used
> for natural resource harvesting and also as a tourist attraction
> to the hot springs and the parks and all of the different beauties
> of the area. So it's a very diverse, hardy sort of a connotation
> to that word.
>
> —Twenty-five-year resident of Appalachia

Imagine two older people meet on a plane, one from Hawaii and the other from West Virginia. They strike up a conversation and eventually the discussion turns to their health. Because they are similar in age, they share some common ailments: stiff muscles, problems remembering important events, and maybe even elevated cholesterol or heart disease. As their conversation continues, one shares concerns about family members who have died from cancer, children who suffer with asthma and diabetes, and grandchildren struggling because of developmental delays. Which of the two travelers do you think is more likely to mention these additional health conditions?

If you think the West Virginian is more likely to experience poor health, you are correct. Hawaii consistently ranks as one of the healthiest states in the country, based on many indicators including obesity rates, mental health, and some environmental conditions. In contrast, West Virginia consistently ranks as one of the least healthy states according to these same indicators.[1] Even if you are not a health professional, you can probably speculate as to why Hawaiians are healthier than West Virginians. Access to health care, genetics, and lifestyle contribute to differences between states, but health is a complicated interaction among multiple forces. Understanding the impacts of poverty, education, and environmental contamination is critical to understanding health. These external forces, or social determinants of health, encompass economic, political, and environmental conditions and contribute to health disparities tied to where people live. Your place of residence, including your country, state, neighborhood, and house, affects your overall health and well-being and differentiates you from others.

Social determinants are the "conditions in the environments in which people are born, live, learn, work, play, worship, and age that affect a wide range of health, functioning, and quality-of-life outcomes and risks."[2] Collectively, these conditions comprise "place," but they go beyond physical geography to include the context of where people live. Social determinants and their connection to place are part of the national dialogue for advancing health and addressing health disparities. The strategic plan for public health in the United States is called *Healthy People*. Every ten years, the US Department of Health and Human Services engages stakeholders to identify long-range goals and near-term objectives for improving the nation's health. *Healthy People 2020* is the third installment of the plan, but the first version to include social determinants of health. Just like the landscape varies from location to location, so do social determinants such as food security, environmental contamination, and community context. We can measure differences in social determinants both globally and locally.

Location and place interact with factors that affect health. Access to public and private health services, an individual's likelihood of being obese, and a community's ability to recover from a major disaster are examples. This being so, I became more interested in the impact of environmental quality on public health. This led me to consider whether some of the unique situations in which Appalachian people live is connected to their health. I knew that the Robert Wood Johnson Foundation has been comparing health among US counties since 2008 using multiple indicators. Its work tells us that, when it comes to life expectancy and overall health, zip code may be as important as genetic code.[3] You may be prone to cancer because of your family history, but your chances of actually getting and dying from cancer increase because of where you live. As many have stated, "heredity loads the gun, environment pulls the trigger."

For better or worse, where people live, work, and play is inextricably tied to their health. To know about their health is to deeply comprehend the place where they live. In a sense, fathoming the connections between health and place portrays the environmental geography of health. Environmental conditions such as contaminated water, unsafe food, poorly designed neighborhoods, polluted air, and inadequate housing characterize places as much as culture, community, and landscape. Why some places are more degraded than others is sometimes easily explained by the assets within their boundaries, as is the case with coal, natural gas, and other energy resources. In these instances, the state of the environment is the result of historical activities tied to cultural and natural resources. In other places, the environment is degraded by political decisions to fulfill short-term economic objectives with little thought to long-term public health consequences.

Both long-term natural resource exploitation and shortsighted decision-making contribute to environmental conditions that threaten the health of Appalachian people. The well-known environmental concerns in the region include devastating mountaintop-removal mining, historic human-caused and natural disasters, ruined streams from untreated sewage, and unhealthy indoor and outdoor air. Not so well-known are how these conditions burden the health of Appalachian people in ways that are disproportionate to other places. This is a missing piece of the Appalachian narrative that begs to be told and was the motivating force for this book. Before delving into stories demonstrating how people are ailing in Appalachian places, let us examine a few key concepts.

THE PLACE CALLED APPALACHIA

A zip code identifies where your house is located on a map, but your place is far more than a zip code. Place includes social, political, cultural, and environmental conditions of the specific location. The concept of place is grounded in geography, identity, childhood, and emotional connectedness.[4] For many of us, a place is meaningful because of both our past experiences and our current circumstances. A place is unique because of the people who inhabit it and the history that defines it. Place means many things; some of them are good, and others not so good. A place can be both hopeful and hopeless, it can both inspire optimism and court despair, and it can both satisfy and frustrate at the same time. Place is complicated but meaningful. Think of the difference between a house and a home. A house has physical boundaries; a home does not. When you think about going home, you may be thinking about your house, but you are also likely to think of your relationships within your community and your experiences there. Your home has shaped who you are; your house is a storage vessel. Home is your place.

Like place, Appalachia has multiple meanings, many of which are not related to map coordinates. Appalachia is defined by its culture, music, food, mountains, and natural resources. Its state and county boundaries "are of no use in defining either the geography or cultural outlines of the region."[5] People who live in the region would agree. Those who call Appalachia home understand it differently than those who do not. This difference contributes to the many negative images of Appalachia in contemporary arts, literature, and media. Unfortunately, these negative portrayals of Appalachian people often overshadow the many positive attributes. For decades, scholars have attempted to more objectively define the region. However, after much debate and discussion, one scholar contends, "we cannot agree on a definition of Appalachia, nor can we definitively say who is Appalachian. Yet we can agree that Appalachia is an important concept because it often makes a difference in people's lives, either personally or as a group."[6]

Because Appalachia has many meanings revolving around place as a social construct, it is almost impossible to imagine drawing precise boundaries of the region. No matter, this is exactly what the federal government did in 1965 when Congress passed the Appalachian Regional Development Act. This legislation created the Appalachian Regional Commission (ARC) and required the ARC to define the boundaries of Appalachia so that government resources could be allotted to the area.[7] The first map included 360 counties within eleven states surrounding the Appalachian Mountains. Over the years, the ARC has obtained congressional approval to expand the region's borders to include 420 counties in thirteen states.

The original map of Appalachia sought to define a region with homogenous socioeconomic and geographic characteristics.[8] Yet as discussions about defining Appalachia have unfolded, we have come to understand that Appalachian people are far from homogenous. We are diverse in countless ways. The current ARC map, which includes counties stretching from western New York through eastern Kentucky and into northeastern Mississippi, indeed reflects this diversity. Even with our diversity, many localities within the region do share similar economic and environmental conditions. High unemployment, low incomes, and persistent poverty concentrate in Appalachia, as do environmental burdens from the past and the present.

Even with its shortfalls, we can still use a map to explore and compare Appalachia to other locations across a range of social, cultural, economic, health, and environmental conditions. A map also conveys a greater understanding about perceptions of this place. When I asked more than three hundred environmental health professionals who work in the region to view the ARC map and state the first word or phrase that came to mind, their responses varied. Many of the responses related to Appalachia's landscape, with words such as "mountains," "wooded," and "rural." Their perceptions of the region went beyond geography and topography, though, and into some societal characteristics, using words such as "poor," "poverty," and "impoverished." Some of the words were compassionate, such as "forgotten" and "heart of America," but others were less so, including "uneducated" and "outcasts."

Almost all the professionals who responded to my survey believe environmental health problems in Appalachia differ from those in other places. At least some of those problems result from political decisions made with promises to improve the economy. In these cases, politicians make unsubstantiated claims that promoting heavy industry and removing the region's natural resources will create jobs. Other environmental problems disproportionately affecting Appalachian people stem from inadequate resources being dedicated to infrastructure, housing, and education. At least some of this inadequacy is tied to tax incentives offered to those companies that politicians promise will solve the region's economic woes. This job-promising-infrastructure-busting situation has played in a loop for decades in Appalachia, but its effect on the environment and public health is often left out of the conversation.

Even as environmental health professionals understand the struggles of Appalachian people when it comes to protecting and improving public health, they agree that something makes this place different than others. They are the ones who inspect landfills, ensure safe food, test water quality, and monitor insects that spread disease. Their mission is to prevent disease by improving the environment, a mission difficult even in wealthy suburbs far from rural Appalachia. These environmental health professionals also understand the challenges of safeguarding public health despite political and economic constraints. Such constraints create underfunded health departments that rely on grants and national politics to set priorities rather than addressing what might be the more important concerns in local places.

For more than fifty years, elected officials at all levels of government have exacerbated problems in the region by politicizing the status of the Appalachian economy. A defining moment came in 1964 when President Lyndon Johnson announced the War on Poverty in his State of the Union speech. His war began in earnest in 1965 when the Appalachian Regional Development Act mandated reducing economic disparities in the region. This mandate is still the ARC's overarching mission. Strategies to address economic disparities largely focus on increasing access to and within the region by building new highways and other transportation infrastructure. While the ARC targets economic disparities with a modicum of gusto and a mound of federal funds, a simmering health crisis is starting to boil over. We see it most alarmingly in the opioid crisis that is gripping Appalachian communities harder than most other places in the country. Opioids may have finally grabbed the attention of politicians, but decades of data reveal that Appalachian people are among the least healthy in the country. There is a vast region in the wealthiest country in the world where nineteenth-century health conditions still exist and even, in some cases, abound.

HEALTH DISPARITIES

There will always be health disparities. People will suffer maladies linked to genetics, gender, and age, and there is nothing we can do about it. Some health disparities are just unavoidable. Other health disparities are systemic and "closely linked with social, economic, and/or environmental disadvantage." These avoidable disparities result from "characteristics historically linked to discrimination or exclusion."[9] Such disparities and so much needless suffering can be prevented through public health strategies and political decisions that prioritize health. Disparities tied to geographic location and socioeconomic status may be invisible, but they are not inevitable.

In a series of reports, the Centers for Disease Control and Prevention (CDC) examines health disparities from a variety of perspectives, including social elements, demographic factors, health care access, and environmental hazards.[10] The CDC specifically connects public health to where people work, how people live, and the economic circumstances of their lives. If the gap between the rich and the poor continues to expand in the United States, avoidable health disparities may get worse even as the overall economy improves. Through a complex set of social, economic, and environmental conditions, poverty increases vulnerability to negative health consequences. Diabetes, malnutrition, occupational injuries, and substance abuse are among the preventable disparities between the rich and the poor. Even as the CDC calls attention to this problem, its work underscores significant gaps in our understanding of place-based health disparities.[11]

When detailing health disparities, the discourse often focuses on people who live within urban areas. For example, in 2015 lead contamination of Flint, Michigan's water supply drew national attention to the plight of low-income people in an urban place. City officials made the decision to switch water sources from Lake Huron to the Flint River despite concerns about their ability to ensure its safety. Almost 45 percent of Flint's residents live in poverty and for more than one year they were exposed to high levels of lead. The Michigan Civil Rights Commission issued a report arguing that the Flint water crisis goes well beyond contemporary technical glitches or political decisions. Rather, they point to a long history of racial injustice and policies that create communities segregated by "race, wealth, and opportunity."[12] Whether blatant or furtive, racial or economic segregation leads to disproportionate environmental exposures in many places, and these exposures lead to avoidable and preventable health outcomes.

In many ways, rural areas exhibit similar health disparities to urban areas. Take asthma, for example. Asthma and other respiratory conditions are not just related to urban air pollution. People in rural areas have asthma but the reasons for it differ in rural Appalachian Pennsylvania from those in inner-city Philadelphia. People may be exposed to similar pollutants in urban and rural areas, but the sources of these pollutants are not the same, so solutions for minimizing exposures are place-specific. Reducing environmental exposures causing asthma in Philadelphia because of urban air pollution requires a different approach than addressing asthma disparities from coal mining activities in the western counties of Appalachian Pennsylvania.

The need for attention to health disparities in rural places is even more critical because of the wide range of contributing factors. There are documented disparities in physical ailments such as diabetes, asthma, and cancer in Appalachia, but Appalachian people also tell us they feel less healthy than most other people in the country.[13] West Virginians on average say they feel in poor health more frequently than people in any other state and this is one reason why it ranks as the least healthy state in the United States[14] This ranking is notable because West Virginia is the only state entirely within the boundaries of Appalachia and is therefore sometimes used as a proxy to represent the region.

Long-term trends in annual surveys suggest that Appalachian people in general are more likely to believe they are in poor health than are residents of other states. When people think they are unhealthy, it is likely they are, even lacking a diagnosis from a health professional. Just the fact that they cannot see a doctor or nurse, for whatever reason, might contribute to how healthy people feel. More objectively, this presumption is supported by the documented lack of access to medical care in Appalachia.[15] The perception of poor health combines with numerous other indicators and is drawing attention to health disparities in a region that has been scrutinized for its economic disparities for a long time.

Since its inception, the Appalachian Regional Commission has worked to reduce, highlight, and document economic disparities. Annually, the ARC classifies, evaluates, and compares employment, poverty, and income within the region and between the region and the rest of the country. Its work underscores the economic struggles that plague Appalachia but does not connect these struggles to public health. The ARC's 2016–20 strategic plan focuses mainly on investing in projects with the potential to improve the economy. Even the one goal in the plan mentioning health does so in the context of creating a "ready workforce" rather than improving public health.[16] The strategic plan notes the existence of health disparities in Appalachia and specifies a need for more investments to improve health status, but focuses on access to services rather than improving environmental conditions or other social determinants.[17]

It is true that lack of access to health care services can exacerbate health disparities, but the rationale for much of the investment in Appalachia has been jobs, not health. Actually detailing health disparities and identifying strategies to reduce them are relatively new endeavors in Appalachia. It wasn't until 1999, more than thirty years after the ARC was formed, that it convened an Appalachian Health Policy Advisory Council to examine health issues. More than two hundred health-related projects were funded by grants running through this council from 2004 through 2010. Most of these were designed to enhance access by constructing facilities and improving equipment. Measurable improvements in access to care in some localities are tied to these projects, but they did not make a discernible impact on reducing health disparities in the region. In 2017, the Robert Wood Johnson Foundation and the ARC collaborated to quantify Appalachian health disparities for the first time. They found that thirty-three out of forty-one health indicators are worse in Appalachia than in the rest of the country.[18]

ENVIRONMENTAL AND HEALTH EQUITY

Understanding health disparities requires more than just identifying differences in health status and access to health care. We can find health disparities in groups who have adequate health care access, so defining good health as good access is much too narrow. The percentage of people with high cholesterol might be higher among middle-class white people who live in the suburbs than low-income African Americans who live in the city. Does this mean that high cholesterol is a health disparity because of these differences between groups? Measles is another compelling health disparity. Even though health officials declared measles eliminated from the United States in 2000, it is coming back. From 2010 to early 2017, the CDC documented more than fifteen hundred cases of measles, mostly in communities where people are unvaccinated.[19] Those who refuse to vaccinate their children because of fear of autism or other health conditions are not poor people in Appalachia. They are generally well-educated, professional white people who, paradoxically, have access to vaccinations because of their income and insurance. Measles is affecting one segment of our population differently than another, but calling this a health disparity confuses and lessens the meaning of the term.

What appears to be a disparity may not be related to the ability to access care. People who get screened are more likely to be diagnosed than those who do not. People who choose not to vaccinate may suffer even though they have ample access to health care resources. Intent and injustice underlie true health disparities and a health disparity is best understood as the "metric that is used to measure progress toward achieving health equity."[20] Health equity embraces social justice as a goal in addressing health disparities. It is based on the principle that all people should be healthy regardless of where they live, how much money they make, or whether they have access to a physician.

Health inequities arise when poverty, education, lack of nutritious food, and environmental quality make some people less healthy than others. They do not exist when people can make choices about their health care, where they live, and the type of work they do. Health inequities also arise when people are unable to afford health screenings, vaccinations, or treatment. There is no inequity when people can pay for prevention and treatment, either through insurance or out-of-pocket, but choose not to partake in either. Not all health disparities are the result of inequities, but those that are tied to place generally are.

Documenting health disparities in Appalachia tends to focus on those that are connected to lifestyle, such as cancer and diabetes, and emphasizes the more controllable individual behaviors rather than uncontrollable living conditions.[21] This attention to addressing behavioral causes of disparities is understandable, since self-reported prevalence of unhealthy behaviors such as smoking is higher in many Appalachian states than others.[22] However, when we zero in on lifestyle we minimize or even disregard the impact of health equity and social justice in creating health disparities.

Just like access to health care, smoking, inactivity, and a poor diet are critical components of health status. Just like access, these behaviors are only part of the story behind health disparities. Additional determinants contribute to overall health, including involuntary exposures, place-based circumstances, and social and environmental conditions. Few have explored the broader relationship between environmental exposures and health outcomes. Those that have, focus on specific environmental circumstances such as mountaintop-removal mining.[23] Some of the poorest people in the United States live in Appalachia, and no one disputes that poverty and health are related. However, in poor communities, living conditions and environmental exposures may be just as important as income, access to health care, and lifestyle. Moreover, people who suffer from poor health because of where they live may have no control over exposures connected to their health status. In some instances, Appalachian people may even create exposures by supporting industries and activities that promise to ease their burden of poverty by providing jobs.

A cyclical relationship exists among poverty, health, and the environment. Therefore, working to improve public health by addressing economic conditions and access to health care without tackling environmental health is incomplete and unsustainable. In at least some instances, exposure to environmental harms is involuntary and based solely on the place in which people live. Even rich people who have access to health care can become sick when exposed to environmental hazards. When groups of people face disproportionate exposures to environmental contaminants simply because of their place of residence, health disparities are the metric for health inequities. Examples of disproportionate environmental exposures are found throughout the United States but some of these exposures are unique in Appalachia and indicate environmental injustice. As evidence mounted that race, and its ties to poverty and place, were important indicators of the location of environmental hazards, the environmental justice movement emerged.

ENVIRONMENTAL JUSTICE

The United Church of Christ (UCC) uncovered relationships between the location of environmentally hazardous sites and race.[24] Its 1987 report, *Toxic Wastes and Race*, was the first to document that urban African American communities are more likely to be exposed to serious environmental hazards than other communities. Twenty years after the 1987 report, the UCC updated its analysis and concluded that not much had changed; race is still an important predictor of exposure to toxic substances.[25] The work by the UCC in urban areas started a national dialogue leading to an executive order from President Bill Clinton. The order requires all federal government agencies to identify and minimize how their decisions could disproportionately affect minority and low-income populations.[26]

Although environmental justice became a mainstream concern in the early 1990s thanks to the efforts of the UCC and others, events in the early 1970s and 1980s in rural Warren County, North Carolina, are considered the historical catalyst for the movement. Warren County borders Virginia and is part of a cluster of counties with the highest percentage of African Americans in the state. This part of North Carolina also has very high poverty rates. In 1973, local people fought against plans to construct a landfill to dispose of polychlorinated biphenyls (PCBs). They were concerned about the possible health consequences of PCBs, which are organic chemicals from previously used electrical transformers, fluorescent light bulbs, oil-based paints, and plastics. PCBs were banned in the United States in 1979 but, because they persist in the environment, managing the disposal of PCB-containing products remains a challenge today.

Warren County residents questioned why the predominantly rural African American community was targeted for the landfill. Protests and confrontations over coal in rural Appalachia have a long history, but the situation in Warren County was different because of the questions it raised about deliberately targeting one community as a dumping site. There were no natural resources or infrastructure in the county that made it the most feasible location for the land-fill. It looked like Warren County was the leading landfill candidate because of its racial composition and high poverty rates, rather than technical factors. In 1982, after almost ten years of resistance, activists successfully blocked the landfill from being built, securing their legacy in the environmental justice movement.

Warren County exemplifies how the official boundaries of the region may mask important contributions of its people. The county is in an Appalachian state, but it is just outside of the ARC-designated boundaries of the region. Warren County might well identify with Appalachia culturally, but it is not con-sidered Appalachia on the map. Regardless, this is an important case because it was a defining moment in environmental justice in America generally and rural America specifically. Warren County scenarios are becoming more prominent in rural Appalachia with contemporary environmental insults such as hydraulic fracturing for natural gas and oil. Every new protest in Appalachia contributes to our understanding of the relationship between place and health and serves to exemplify how local people are speaking out about projects with questionable economic benefits and unquestionable and inequitable environmental harms.

Unfortunately, in some instances, residents in rural Appalachian commu-nities contribute to projects that create harmful environmental exposures. In places with persistently bad economic conditions, communities may support any kind of development offering the potential for quick economic returns, especially if jobs are on the table. This support abounds even if the relief is certain to be temporary and almost always intensifies the debate between ad-vocates of environment protection versus economic development. Some of the stories I tell in this book underscore difficult choices Appalachian people face when both environmental health and economic impacts are uncertain but jobs are promised. Much in the way the UCC report highlights disparities in urban areas, I seek to highlight some of the unique aspects of rural Appalachia that exacerbate environmental injustices, health inequities, and health disparities. I also draw attention to the important role of and challenges for environmental and public health policymakers and professionals as they pursue solutions to place-based inequities and health disparities.

THE PLACE OF ENVIRONMENTAL AND PUBLIC HEALTH

Public health is both a profession and a mission. The profession includes personnel at multiple governmental levels, often partnering with business, nongovernmental organizations, and researchers. The mission of public health is "the fulfillment of society's interest in assuring the conditions in which people can be healthy."[27] Public health professionals create and implement strategies to stop disease and injury from spreading through populations. Public health is easily distinguishable from medical care because of its attention to prevention rather than treatment. Also, different than medical care, the patient in public health is an entire community, not one single individual. The more than one-hundred-year history of public health success represents its key role in improving the nation's health and suggests new challenges moving forward.

In 1900, the leading causes of death in the United States were pneumonia, tuberculosis, and diarrhea. At the end of the twentieth century, a strong and valued public health system was able to minimize or, in some cases, eliminate many infectious diseases.[28] Antibiotics and medical care strategies for treating individuals are only part of the reason for the decline in infectious diseases throughout the century. Interrupting the way pathogens move from person to person, or the mode of transmission, is just as important as preventive drugs and individual patient treatments. Air, food, water, or vectors such as mosquitoes and ticks are needed for some of the most infectious diseases to spread. Tackling these modes of transmission is the crux of environmental health and many significant historical public health achievements are the direct result of environmental health practices. Examples include water and wastewater sanitation, food safety protocols, hazardous waste management, and outdoor and indoor air quality control. There is no doubt that attention to environmental conditions in specific places decreases the burden of disease.

As society transitioned into the twenty-first century, public health priorities changed dramatically. Now, the United States is largely comprised of places where chronic conditions such as heart disease and cancers are the leading causes of death. These chronic illnesses feed a massive health care system that amplifies the role of prescription drugs and high-cost treatments. Chronic diseases also shift the structural elements of environmental health from straightforward approaches such as disinfecting tap water, removing lead from gasoline, and banning specific pesticides. There are clear environmental solutions to persistent health problems such as obesity, asthma, and some cancers, but they are muddled by politics, economics, and history.

Environmental health actions to prevent chronic disease involve global, national, and local strategies to improve living conditions and the political will to do so. These are place-based actions and numerous organizations at all levels of government complicate implementing these actions. Public health responsibilities are housed in large federal departments in Washington, state departments of health and the environment, and small county health departments such as those in the remote corners of Appalachia. Public health in the federal government involves a morass of agencies, institutions, organizations, and offices. In some cases, multiple units within one federal department compete for resources to address a single public health issue. Ultimately, if local resources are limited by structural inequities, programs and policies at the federal level may have very little impact on the wholesomeness of your next bite of food, the cleanliness of your next glass of water, or the clarity of your next breath of air.

Some of the most vital public health infrastructure is localized in county and city health departments across the country. These local agencies identify and address place-based environmental health priorities. Local health departments are funded by a patchwork of sources that include federal and state subsidies, governmental and foundation grants, and local taxes. This means that they are often hamstrung by uncertain and unsustainable resources. The restrictive funding of local health agencies is an example of a structural inequity that contributes to health disparities. Some of the people in greatest need of preventive services live in places, including Appalachia, without adequate local public health support.

Just as there are barriers to primary care services in many Appalachian places, public health services are also out of reach. Resource constraints are critical blockades to implementing the mission of public health, especially considering that it is tricky to document the benefits of prevention. We can easily tally up the costs of prevention in dollars spent on programs such as restaurant inspections and spraying for mosquitoes. It is much more difficult to put a monetary value on the lives saved and illnesses averted through these types of programs. One result of the complexity of detailing benefits in monetary terms goes back to the emphasis on prioritizing economic development over public health. It is straightforward to itemize the presence of new jobs, but difficult to itemize the absence of disease. This is a message that I will return to numerous times throughout this book.

Local governments in rural Appalachia often face major resource hurdles in implementing and sustaining public health programs. These hurdles intensify existing health disparities by exacerbating challenges in preventing acute illnesses as well as chronic health conditions. As an example, there are underlying factors contributing to diabetes and obesity. Public health officials identify obesity as a major public health issue in America, going as far as calling it an epidemic.[29] But what about the underlying factors contributing to obesity? Researchers have successfully linked genetics and lifestyle to obesity, but clearly there are other factors contributing to the epidemic. Searching for these factors has led to an expanding field in public health generally referred to as addressing the built environment, which understands that place is a critical determinant of health. It also means that successfully preventing obesity and its associated health conditions requires broader measures than only targeting internal forces such as lifestyle. To make the greatest impact, we must address external forces such as land-use planning and community design.

I write about Appalachian populations who face health disparities because of *where* they live, rather than *how* they live. Such a place-based approach is the very foundation for the pursuit of environmental justice by minimizing exposure inequities that lead to health disparities.

STRUCTURE OF THE BOOK

There are documented disparities in cancers, asthma, diabetes, substance abuse, and many other health conditions in Appalachia. Answering the question of why these disparities persist even as other places in the country get healthier requires us to investigate many factors, including where people live. This means that we need to explore environmental health differences tied to specific places. We also need to probe into the reasons for these differences, paying attention to controllable inequities that contribute to them. In this book I describe some of what is currently known about environmental exposures and health disparities in Appalachia. I do not intend this work to be a comprehensive account of the relationship between the environment and health in the region. I also do not claim that all the information I present in the following pages is new; I did not gather primary data about environmental exposures, for instance. Rather, I hope to contribute a perspective in which place-based conditions are seen as at least part of the reason why Appalachian people are among the least healthy Americans. Many of these conditions are out of our control, because they are either born from a history of environmental abuse or are subject to current constraints leading to environmental neglect.

To paint a picture of the impact of environmental health disparities in Appalachia I use published research, information from interviews, and personal observations. My intent is twofold. First, I strive to provide the reader with verifiable data related to specific environmental conditions. There is a wealth of available statistics for comparing counties in Appalachia to the rest of the country, and the map of the region is essential to make these comparisons. Second, I highlight specific Appalachian places as examples of communities that are exposed to environmental conditions unique to the region.

Before diving into specific stories, I lay the foundation for environmental health in chapter 1. This foundation is critical to framing the remainder of the book because I define environmental health and examine possible inequities in implementing strategies to reduce risks in Appalachia places. I summarize environmental health infrastructure at the global, national, and local levels to provide some context for the challenges and circumstances in Appalachia.

The built environment is a significant public health issue especially when it comes to inequities that contribute to health disparities. A great deal of attention to the health impacts of the built environment revolves around understanding rising obesity rates relative to community design. The rate of obesity in Appalachia is higher than the national average, but the reasons for these rates are more complicated than the way communities are designed. Other health disparities in Appalachia are clearly tied to land-use decisions in rural areas. There are disproportionate environmental exposures in Appalachia arising from both inside and outside living conditions. By comparing Appalachian to non-Appalachian communities in chapter 2, I highlight prevailing inequities in exposures to radon, lead, and secondhand smoke and the health disparities these exposures cause.

The old coal camps serving as home to some rural Appalachian people have many of the most basic environmental health problems. It is hard to imagine that there are still people in the United States who do not have access to safe drinking water, but places throughout Appalachia lack such critical infrastructure. A major chemical spill in the drinking-water source for Charleston, West Virginia, accentuated the consequences of failing regulatory and technical infrastructure. Ensuring safe water is a main environmental health function, but private systems predominate in rural Appalachia and are problems in communities, such as coal camps and company towns, that were not intended to be places of long-term habitation. Chapter 3 draws attention to public and private drinking-water supplies and wastewater treatment systems, explaining the difference between them and documenting specific instances of contamination and inequitable exposures in Appalachia.

Like drinking water, food safety affects everyone, and its health impacts are usually completely preventable. Multistate outbreaks regularly occur in the

United States and the CDC estimates that more than 48 million Americans suffer foodborne illness every year. On the other hand, food security is more localized and targets the poor. The documented health impacts of food insecurity include diabetes and obesity, both of which are at epidemic levels in Appalachia. Chapter 4 describes specific food safety and security issues in the region and offers examples of programs and policies aimed at improving these conditions. The number of farmers' markets is expanding and is touted as a major part of the strategy to tackle food insecurity. However, in chapter 4, I examine the uncertain impact of farmers' markets on this critical issue in Appalachia.

Water quality and food security are usually localized problems. On the other hand, pollution emitted from industry and waste facilities affects broader areas throughout Appalachia. Some places in the region are assaulted by multiple pollutants to their water and air, exposing local people to a range of potential health effects. At least some of these exposures are because facilities were built in Appalachia even though other locations might have been more technically sound choices. Chapter 5 highlights exposures to chemicals and other pollutants arising, at least in part, from political motives to bring jobs to the region. The region seems to be ground zero for solving the nation's energy needs. Addressing these needs without the foresight to understand the potential public health impacts is a recurring scenario in Appalachia, one which will never address economic disparities in a sustainable way.

Evidence of Appalachia's role in energy supply is found in its thousands of natural gas wells. In some ways, shale gas development in the form of hydraulic fracturing resembles coal mining in the early twentieth century. Appalachian communities are again providing energy for the nation while being burdened with legacy environmental health problems. A major concern with hydraulic fracturing is the lack of research related to potential public health risks from both the drilling itself and managing waste arising from the process. Nevertheless, drilling is proceeding at a rapid pace in Appalachia because of both the natural resources and economic conditions in the region. In chapter 6, I explore shale gas development and other extractive industries, including coal. I draw attention to health disparities that we have now documented with coal mining but have yet to document with hydraulic fracturing.

Activities to remove natural resources from Appalachia sometimes have disastrous consequences. Regrettably, both human-caused and weather-related disasters are commonplace. Some of the most memorable and historic natural disasters, such as floods, have plagued the region along with equally historic "unnatural" disasters such as coal-ash spills. Appalachian people are also vulnerable to predicted impacts from climate change because of a lack of infrastructure and resources, but they may be more resilient thanks to their history with disasters. Some climate change projections suggest improvements in specific environmental conditions in the region, but I explain in chapter 7 that there is a connection between climate change and disasters in Appalachia. Even though people in the region have endured many significant disasters in the past, climate change is likely to be a game changer. I feature some of these disasters in this chapter to weigh Appalachia's vulnerability to projections about the future of extreme weather events.

When writing about Appalachia, it is essential to offer the narrative in a way that is relevant to those who live here. One way I attempt to do this is to begin each chapter with a quote from an Appalachian resident or local environmental health professional, to offer the perspectives of people who live and work in the region. After sifting through several years of interviews, focus groups, and surveys, I chose relevant and impactful passages. To further contextualize the issues raised in this book and to add a human element to each chapter, stories of specific places serve as examples of some of the unique environmental exposures existing in Appalachia. These stories were recommended by numerous people during background interviews for this project. In almost every case, I visited the places I write about and talked to people in the area.

A note on terminology: Throughout the book, I use "environmental health" to identify both environmental exposures and conditions affecting public health, and to identify the profession that seeks to minimize these exposures. On the other hand, "public health" is more broadly used than "environmental health." Exposures affecting public health include those that are behavior-based, such as smoking and eating a poor diet. Environmental health may be narrower in focus than public health, but it is the key to reducing many health disparities because it is the first line of defense in improving health status.

1

Foundations of Environmental Health

County health departments in Appalachia have perpetually suffered from a lack of resources and populations there are often underserved.

—Appalachian environmental health professional

Because public health issues have changed dramatically since the early 1900s our job (should) involve a more proactive approach than in years past. Gone are the days when we can just administer a vaccine. Diabetes, heart disease and obesity are the big public health issues yet we continue to address the more traditional issues (which are still important) like water and sewage, food handler sanitation and vector issues.

—Appalachian environmental health professional

ENVIRONMENTAL HEALTH AFFECTS EVERYONE EVERY DAY. This phrase defines the impact of environmental health programs and professionals on society. As a prominent component of public health practice, environmental health prevents disease and promotes health by controlling and minimizing environmental exposures. Those of us who live in developed countries are generally more concerned about chronic conditions such as heart disease and diabetes, rather than diarrhea and malaria because of environmental health. We breathe clean air, eat safe food, and drink clean water because of environmental health. Under current climatic conditions, we are relatively safe from deadly diseases spread by mosquitoes and other vectors because of environmental health. We can also feel confident that we will not contract a blood-borne disease while we are getting a tattoo or a haircut because of environmental health. When there is a disaster such as a hurricane or flood, we are likely to suffer only minor health impacts and recover relatively quickly because of environmental health.

ENVIRONMENTAL HEALTH: PAST TO PRESENT

For centuries, we have relied on environmental health practices to ensure conditions conducive to good health, practices that we can trace all the way back to ancient Rome. As Rome's population was growing, so was the amount of human waste. Raw sewage not only made the city stink, it also threatened its drinking water. Just like a major modern city, the inability to provide safe drinking water jeopardized ancient Rome's growth, even though there was a clean water source in the vicinity. Imagine the scene in 300 BC in which officials in Rome were discussing how to transport water from nearby mountains into the city. Ultimately, they built a system of aqueducts that used gravity to move clean water into Rome and dirty water out of it. These early environmental engineers laid the foundation for modern water systems and established the importance of solving environmental problems to safeguard health and improve communities. The Roman aqueducts promoted the city's growth and demonstrate historical connections among planning, environmental protection, and public health. In a sense, environmental health was born when water started flowing through the aqueducts.

The first environmental health professionals sought to limit the spread of disease by improving living conditions, protecting environmental assets, and controlling modes of transmission. In this profession, the environment includes microlevel settings, such as houses, restaurants, and institutions, as well as macrolevel surroundings such as outdoor air, neighborhoods, and occupational situations. Although the ancient Roman aqueducts exemplify historical environmental health, the profession only became organized in the mid-1800s.

One of the earliest documented gatherings dedicated to understanding and controlling environmental factors to improve health was held in the middle of the nineteenth century.[1] At the first in a series of International Sanitary Conferences convened in 1851, health officials and experts discussed how to control the spread of cholera.[2] Cholera was killing thousands of people every day and threatening economic progress in some of the most vibrant cities in the world, including New York City. Even though health professionals did not understand the cause of cholera at the time of the first meeting, there was clear understanding of the importance of stopping the spread of the disease and by reducing potential environmental exposures.

Public health experts and diplomats at these conferences also discussed plague and yellow fever. We now know that these two diseases are spread by insect vectors—fleas for the former and mosquitoes for the latter. In the years leading up to the first conference, cholera, yellow fever, and plague were rampant across the world. Conference attendees promoted the role of hygiene and sanitation to curtail the disease, specifically focusing on using quarantine as a preventive measure. There are not many records of the months-long first conference, but it failed in making any significant progress in controlling cholera. However, it brought attention to the connection between public health and economic health and laid the foundation for international collaboration. The sanitary conferences focused on water- and vector-borne diseases, two major components of modern-day environmental health. Of the maladies that motivated international problem solving, cholera defines the environmental health profession.

Cholera's central role in the history of environmental health began in 1849 when John Snow, a London anesthesiologist, argued that it could be spread from person to person and that there was an environmental source. In his detailed and somewhat gory description of the symptoms of cholera, he notes that not everyone who encounters sick people will become ill. He also details the impact that social status and living conditions have on the spread of cholera: "It is amongst the poor, where the whole family live, sleep, cook, eat, and wash in a single room, that cholera has been found to spread when once introduced, and still more in those places termed common lodging-houses, in which several families were crowded into a single room. It was amongst the vagrant class, who lived in this crowded state, that cholera was most fatal in 1832. . . When, on the other hand, cholera is introduced into the better kinds of houses, ... it hardly ever spreads from one family member to the other."[3]

Snow explains that miners suffered the most in Great Britain during this time period. Working conditions in the mines allowed for little personal hygiene throughout the day and exposed miners to open defecation. It was clear that living and working conditions contributed to cholera's impact. However, Snow also noted that cholera was spreading in the absence of person-to-person contact and in areas with relatively good sanitation facilities. After extensive data-gathering, he concluded that people were being exposed to cholera in their drinking water. His conclusion was not fully accepted by politicians and many other medical professionals until the 1880s, after another physician identified a microorganism shaped like a comma as the cause of cholera.

Snow's connection between drinking water and cholera cases is among the most important historical moments in environmental health.[4] As the disease decimated entire families and neighborhoods, many health officials, politicians, and engineers were clinging to the belief that something in the air, called "miasma," was causing the epidemics. Snow, on the other hand, used a basic geographic information system—he drew a map of cases and deaths—to deduce a relationship between the location of a single drinking-water pump and the disease in one London neighborhood. After Snow convinced the politicians to remove the handle from the pump, cholera cases in the neighborhood dropped, and environmental epidemiology was born. Environmental health grew from this discovery of a place-based exposure that caused human illness.

The cholera epidemics framed discussions at all the International Sanitary Conferences throughout the early twentieth century. These conferences facilitated the creation of the World Health Organization (WHO) in 1948. The WHO explicitly defines health as "a state of complete physical, mental and social well-being and not merely the absence of disease or infirmity."[5] The WHO also focused on the health of populations rather than individuals and thus institutionalized public health globally. In public health, groups of people, rather than individuals, are the patients. In public health, prevention, rather than treatment, is the strategy. Public health professionals believe in the saying that an ounce of prevention is worth a pound of cure. There is little question that it is more effective to prevent rather than treat disease. It is more economical to society for people to eat healthier than suffer from heart conditions, and smoking cessation programs are less expensive than treating individuals for lung cancer. The most efficient way to deal with health conditions that are spread from environmental contact is to stop the exposures in the first place.

It is almost impossible to think of a single health outcome that would be more cost-effective to treat than prevent. However, public health often appears expensive since it involves policies that engage entire populations, whether at the global, national, state, or local levels. While the costs seem insurmountable, the benefits of prevention are difficult to quantify. You cannot count the number of people who did not become sick or die because of a specific intervention. Furthermore, the burden of cost falls on local places, often in the form of taxes. This means that low-income communities struggle to pay for public health just like low-income individuals struggle to pay for health care. In tying preventive public health programs to local taxes, we have created a system that contributes to inequities that lead to health disparities. Even with its long history of successfully preventing disease, environmental health is often among the first local public health programs eliminated during times of austerity. When a local health department has a range of mandates to deliver, including vaccinating children, providing nutritional programs, and offering an array of nursing and health care services, inspecting restaurants or trapping mosquitoes may seem dispensable.

Local health departments are on the front lines of environmental health practice, thus tying environmental health to place. Overall, environmental health is a place-based profession and there are multiple local, state, national, and international agencies and organizations responsible for it. In this chapter, I provide an overview of environmental health and focus on how organizations at all levels are taking steps to address health disparities connected to environmental exposures and inequities. My purpose is to provide an orientation to the profession as an important framework for exploring environmental health in Appalachia.

ENVIRONMENTAL HEALTH: GLOBAL TO LOCAL

Because "environment" is broadly defined to include physical as well as social factors, the profession is diverse, addressing problems ranging from childhood lead poisoning to climate change. To be an environmental health practitioner you must have general knowledge in chemistry, physics, mathematics, microbiology, and epidemiology. Environmental health professionals prevent illness and injury caused by food, swimming pools, wastewater, drinking water, solid and hazardous waste, disease vectors (e.g., insects, rodents), and indoor and outdoor air quality. In addition, they address noise pollution, occupational safety and health, radiation, disaster and emergency preparedness, and environmental health in institutional and other built environments. The breadth of the field means that environmental health maintains the health and well-being of the public every day.

Those in the profession share a common goal of minimizing exposures to prevent disease and injuries. Tactics to accomplish this goal are somewhat convoluted and fragmented, and can involve international, national, state, and local governments working with varying degrees of cohesion. Environmental health laws and policies can be found in international treaties, national and state statutes, and local ordinances. Nonregulatory programs that include technical assistance, land-use planning, and health education are also found in multiple agencies from international organizations to local health departments. Much of the profession either directly or indirectly participates in issues surrounding health disparities and inequities, with some organizations specifically focusing on the environmentally related social determinants of health.

Global Environmental Health

Among the international organizations with roles in environmental health are the World Health Organization, its regional office the Pan American Health Organization, and the United Nations Environment Programme. These organizations monitor global disease, work to minimize conditions that create unhealthy populations, and communicate the status of public health to multiple audiences extending from national governments to individuals. The most pressing global public health issues are often connected to environmental health. Well-known examples of these include the malaria parasite and the Zika virus, which are spread by mosquitoes, the waterborne polio virus, and the Ebola virus, which is likely associated with bats. Even though some of the most significant global public health threats are not currently of concern in many developed countries, environmental health issues such as food safety and access to clean drinking water are.

The WHO has been the most prominent international agency when it comes to preventing diseases and protecting public health. The United Nations created the WHO in 1948 by combining several international health agencies. The World Health Assembly, which oversees the WHO, is composed of representatives from UN member states. This assembly meets annually to set policies, review global health trends, and develop priorities. Reducing health disparities and addressing the needs of vulnerable populations are significant areas of focus of the WHO. Its environmental initiatives target climate change, food safety, air pollution, and water sanitation. The WHO highlighted the potential impacts of social determinants on health disparities at the World Conference on Social Determinants of Health in 2011. In 2012, the World Health Assembly endorsed the Rio Political Declaration on Social Determinants of Health, which focuses on reducing the root causes of health inequities, including by improving "daily living conditions."[6] These daily living conditions are place-based and include food security, safe drinking water, and wastewater sanitation.

The WHO identifies people who are most vulnerable to suffering from a lack of attention to or resources for environmental health. For example, even though there has been progress in gaining worldwide access to clean drinking water, there are "stark disparities across regions, between urban and rural areas, and between the rich and the poor and marginalized."[7] As developing countries grow, public health impacts from unsafe water grow as well. As much as 90 percent of wastewater in the most populated coastal cities flows untreated into adjacent bodies of water.[8] This means massive amounts of raw sewage contaminate oceans, rivers, and lakes and increase the likelihood of pathogens spreading from place to place. After more than one hundred years of effort and attention, cholera is still endemic in many countries and epidemics occur with frightening regularity. The persistence of cholera serves as an example of a global environmental health inequity that disproportionately affects the poor and those who live in places without resources to deal with water contamination.

Global inequities also exist in exposures to air pollution, susceptibility to food insecurity, and vulnerability to the potential public health impacts from climate change. However, this is hardly a definitive account of worldwide environmental health inequities. Poverty is a leading social determinant that translates these inequities into health disparities. In rural communities in developing countries, simply preparing a meal creates a significant health risk from indoor cooking stoves. The indoor air pollutants generated from these stoves are of concern to the WHO because three billion people still use wood and charcoal to cook inside their homes.[9] The stoves create unhealthy levels of multiple pollutants and result in millions of avoidable deaths and illnesses every year. In addition, the black carbon created during cooking further contributes to localized air pollution as well as global greenhouse gas emissions.

The WHO is currently the leading global public health organization, but the Pan American Health Organization (PAHO) is considered the oldest international public health agency. Diseases spread through the environment stimulated the creation of PAHO in 1902. A cross-governmental Pan American Sanitary Code was ratified in 1924. The code specifies that countries will notify others of the status of specific diseases such as cholera, typhus, yellow fever, and smallpox and lays out objectives and protocols for controlling disease. The PAHO identifies the code as the "greatest achievement in health policy-making in the American hemisphere."[10] The PAHO's 2014–19 strategic plan draws attention to "persistent health inequities between and within countries."[11] Addressing social determinants of health is critical to the PAHO's mission and the strategic plan "mainstreams" social determinants into all "policies, programs, and projects." PAHO collaborates with the WHO and other international organizations such as the United Nations Environment Programme (UNEP) on major environmental health projects.

The UNEP is directly affiliated with the United Nations since it is led by an under-secretary-general. It is the lead international environmental organization with a mission dedicated to sustainability. One of its main roles is to educate governments and the public about the connection between the environment and health. Since 2005, the UNEP has been involved in a Poverty-Environment Initiative (PEI) focused on making the poverty-environment connection a factor in decision-making at all levels of government. The underlying philosophy for the PEI is that the environment is "closely linked to the livelihoods, health and vulnerability of every inhabitant of the world and specifically for people living in poverty."[12] The PEI promotes tools to alleviate poverty and improve environmental conditions in conjunction with enhancing economies in developing countries.

Global health organizations and initiatives contextualize the determinants of health disparities found across the world. In many ways, how global environmental health actors describe the plight of poor communities is strikingly similar to how it is described in some places in Appalachia. For example, in highlighting conditions in Nairobi's slums, the WHO identifies key factors that contribute to poor health: inadequate and poor access to health services, unhealthy lifestyles and unstable social structures, and insecurity and neglect. These types of similarities have led to perceptions of Appalachia as being part of America's "Third World," a label many in Appalachia resent. While it is true that there are similar environmental problems, the documented place-based health inequities in Appalachia are more perplexing than those in countries without the resources of the United States.

There is fresh emphasis on addressing environmental conditions as important social determinants of health, especially at the international level. Specific attention is paid to vulnerable populations in developing countries. Even the international organizations recognize that there are inequitable exposures within countries, not just between countries. While some lament the plight of the poor in developing countries, we tend to overlook health inequities in our own country. Some also subscribe to the notion that poor people are mainly unhealthy because of individual lifestyle and behavioral choices rather than because of localized exposures tied to place. That environmental and health inequities tied to place and socioeconomic status exist in rich, industrialized countries such as the United States is alarming and unjustifiable.

The reason that the poverty-environment relationship is such a powerful indicator of health is that poverty transcends more than just differences in the wealth of individuals or households. It also affects community wealth and interferes with the ability of environmental health professionals to do their jobs. Investigating and examining poverty and environmental interactions in local American communities should be approached with the same respect and concern as it is globally. There are environmental inequities throughout America leading to health disparities, and these inequities are amplified by an often-inadequate approach to local environmental health.

National Environmental Health

There are four lines of defense against disease: environmental and public health, immunity, lifestyle, and medical care. Environmental health is the first line of defense because it is a preventive, cost-effective, and efficient approach to protecting public health—when adequate resources are available. Unfortunately, the long-standing US approach to health policy ranks individual medical treatment over large-scale prevention. Many find it distressing that we focus so much on treating individual patients at the expense of population-based public health approaches, because prevention is likely to make a bigger difference on controlling some chronic and communicable diseases.[13]

Public health professionals were cautiously optimistic as the treatment-based approach to health care started to shift somewhat with the 2010 Affordable Care Act (ACA), also known as "Obamacare." The ACA created a fund for public health and required insurers to cover specific preventive services.[14] The ACA has been controversial because elected officials, rather than public health or health care professionals, are making decisions about how best to deal with the nation's health. As politicians discuss changes to legislation, they create volatility in the health care system, compounding instability in public health services.

In the United States, resources for improving and maintaining public health are "unpredictable, inadequate, and uncoordinated."[15] We are reminded of the accuracy of this assessment on a regular basis as multistate outbreaks of food-borne illness continue to rise every year, Ebola arrives in the country, and the Zika virus spreads from state to state. Even though the laws that govern public health practice are comprehensive and some strong regulations are in place, many places lack the resources to fully implement and enforce regulations. Politicians further jeopardize public health and risk widening health disparities when they prioritize deregulation and champion more local control of environmental protection. Local control may seem like a valid approach to addressing place-based environmental health, but it amplifies vulnerability in the most impoverished communities because of persistent resource limitations.

Local resource constraints are intensified by the multifaceted, complicated, and "uncoordinated" approach to developing, implementing, and enforcing public health protections. At least part of the problem with effectively addressing health in America is that there are so many departments, agencies, and organizations involved. Overall, environmental health is one of the most disjointed components of the US government, largely because there are numerous players with seemingly distinct roles even though they are in overlapping programs. These components range from departments that are part of the president's cabinet to small ad-hoc advisory committees associated with specific environmental health issues.

There are currently fifteen departments represented in the president's cabinet, and at least nine of them include aspects of environmental health. Environmental responsibilities are found in the Departments of Health and Human Services (DHHS); Homeland Security (DHS); Energy; Transportation; Housing and Urban Development (HUD); Labor; Commerce; Agriculture (USDA); and the Interior. DHHS and USDA have the most extensive portfolio of environmental health activities among the cabinet-level departments. DHHS is the primary agency responsible for public health, including environmental health. DHHS includes the Centers for Disease Control and Prevention (CDC), the Agency for Toxic Substances and Disease Registry (ATSDR), the Food and Drug Administration, the National Institutes of Health (NIH), and the Indian Health Service. All the components of DHHS house crucial environmental health programs, such as the National Center for Environmental Health (NCEH) in the CDC and the National Institute of Environmental Health Sciences (NIEHS) in the NIH.

With a few exceptions, the agencies and institutes within the DHHS are not significantly involved in enforcing environmental laws and regulations. Rather, DHHS plays a critical role in coordinating disease surveillance, investigating outbreaks, conducting research, and funding state and local governments through grants and contracts. For example, the mission of the NIEHS is "to discover how the environment affects people in order to promote healthier lives."[16] The institute fulfills this mission through major internal research initiatives, grants for external research, and training and education programs for environmental health practice. One of the goals of the 2018–23 NIEHS Strategic Plan is to uncover "the exposure burdens that combine with other social determinants of health, such as age, gender, education, race, and income, to create health disparities, as well as working to ensure environmental justice."[17]

On the other hand, the USDA is heavily involved in enforcement, particularly when it comes to food safety. Under the umbrella of the USDA, the Agricultural Marketing Service works with farmers' markets, the Animal and Plant Health Inspection Service monitors and regulates the health of animals that are food sources, and the Food Safety Inspection Service is responsible for ensuring the safety of meat, poultry, and processed eggs. Inspectors from the USDA have an almost impossible job protecting the nation's food supply. They have thousands of facilities to regulate in the face of dwindling resources and burgeoning demands from an ever-changing food industry.[18]

The Department of Homeland Security is the newest cabinet-level department, having been created in response to the attacks on September 11, 2001. DHS manages federal disaster response, such as addressing and responding to shelter, water, and safety issues that may arise after a hurricane. The Federal Emergency Management Agency (FEMA) and the US Coast Guard are in DHS and prepare for and respond to disasters. In addition, the Health Threats Resilience Division in DHS monitors potential health threats from infectious agents that could be used in a bioterrorism attack and threaten national security. The BioWatch Program in this division involves state environmental and public health agencies in air monitoring to detect potential bioterrorism attacks.

The Departments of Housing and Urban Development and Labor also have some environmental health responsibilities. HUD influences the built environment through many of its funding programs that are set up to improve living conditions for lower-income Americans. The Department of Labor is responsible for workplace and occupational safety to prevent death, illness, and injury on the job. The Department of Labor also houses the Bureau of Labor Statistics, which is an important and influential source of information about health determinants such as unemployment, earnings, and occupation as well as other economic indicators that indirectly influence health.

These cabinet departments constitute one aspect of environmental health at the federal level. Independent agencies such as the Environmental Protection Agency and quasi-governmental groups and commissions play major roles in environmental and public health protection as well. Other federal noncabinet authorities related to environmental health include

- the Consumer Product Safety Commission, which is responsible for recalls of products that could injure, sicken, or kill people;

- the Federal Mine Safety and Health Review Commission, which reviews cases related to hazards in mining;

- the National Science Foundation, which funds research related to environmental exposures and health outcomes;

- the Occupational Safety and Health Administration, which oversees workplaces to minimize injury and death on the job;

- the Nuclear Regulatory Commission, which is responsible for licensing and regulating nuclear power plants in the United States; and

- the Tennessee Valley Authority, a corporation owned by the US government that makes decisions related to electricity generation, energy policy, and environmental issues related to these.

It is likely that the EPA is the primary agency that comes to mind when thinking about the US government's role in environmental health. The EPA is the central US governmental entity in environmental health because it regulates pollution, provides technical assistance to states, and conducts research about the health effects of chemicals and other agents. Federal environmental laws and regulations addressing air and water pollution, waste management, pesticide use, and climate change are among the important mandates of the EPA.

Because the administrator of the EPA is not a member of the president's cabinet, he or she might not have direct access to the administration like the department secretaries do. On the other hand, the importance of the EPA varies from administration to administration, so the impact of the administrator varies as well. Ever since President Richard Nixon created the EPA, legislators, presidents, environmental groups, and others have discussed and debated elevating its head to a cabinet position. These efforts took on new urgency during the administration of President George H. W. Bush and have continued in subsequent administrations amid concerns over the potential for weakening environmental protection. As in the case of the Department of Homeland Security in 2001, it requires an act of Congress to create a new department led by a secretary.

The need to protect the country from terrorists in the wake of the September 11th attacks galvanized Congress to demonstrate its resolve. In creating DHS, it reworked some of the country's disaster-response infrastructure into one new department, a move that was largely a political exercise. Creating a Department of Environmental Protection would be more politically controversial than doing the same for homeland security, so it is unlikely that this will happen anytime soon. As a matter of fact, during recent presidential campaigns, rhetoric focused instead on eliminating the EPA altogether, much to the dismay of environmental health professionals. Whether or not we see a cabinet-level appointment as symbolic only, it is possible that the lack of cabinet status reflects the lack of US commitment to environmental protection.

Even though the EPA is a major player among all the federal government entities when it comes to environmental health initiatives, the US Public Health Service (USPHS), currently located in DHHS, is probably the most influential for health because it is directly involved in preventing human disease. The origins of the USPHS go back to the late eighteenth and early nineteenth centuries with organized efforts to ensure the health of naval personnel. The navy developed several marine hospitals and appointed a "supervising surgeon" to oversee these facilities. Congress built on the military traditions to establish the USPHS Commissioned Corps in 1889. In 1912, environmental health became an important mandate of this uniformed service as Congress enacted legislation to include sanitation, water supplies, and sewage disposal as part of its responsibilities. The supervising surgeon is now known as the surgeon general and the Commissioned Corps includes environmental health professionals as well as nurses, physicians, dieticians, and numerous other health professionals. Corps members wear the navy uniform and work to prevent the spread of disease related to such events as disasters, outbreaks, and epidemics.

The USPHS and other federal departments and agencies are critical components of the environmental health infrastructure in America. In most cases their roles are national in scope, addressing broad public health concerns that involve multiple states. The federal government also has some direct involvement in local environmental issues, especially when states do not have adequate resources, or the political will, to write and enforce environmental health regulations. Under many landmark state environmental laws, states have the primary authority, or primacy, to enforce regulations that are at least as stringent as federal law. States cannot maintain their primacy without local environmental health professionals, who are the frontline personnel implementing key programs. The local government role in environmental health is constrained by available resources at multiple levels of government. This makes the economic status of communities, counties, and states a key factor in the ability of local public health agencies to be effective. Resource limitations contribute to environmental health inequities and health disparities. Places facing the greatest economic hardship are more likely to struggle with maintaining a safe and healthy environment, and Appalachia is one such place.

Appalachian Environmental Health

The international and national environmental health infrastructure provides context for discussing state and local programs and policies. State governments set environmental health priorities in compliance with broad federal laws while keeping an eye on the local economic impact of these laws. Federal laws are translated into more specific regulations that are enforced and implemented locally. Even though all states comply with the same federal laws, there is not a one-size-fits-all approach when it comes to applying them. Most states tackle environmental health issues similarly to the federal government, with substructures of multiple agencies responsible for specific programs. Not all states have discrete divisions or bureaus responsible for all the topics covered in this book.[19] State governments also work closely with local health departments and agencies, further complicating the public health infrastructure.

In many states, environmental health programs are divided between an agency with a specific mission to protect public health and an agency that focuses on environmental protection. All thirteen Appalachian states have at least one agency dedicated to public health, but they are identified and organized differently. In Alabama, Pennsylvania, Ohio, and Tennessee, the Department of Health is the primary public health agency. South Carolina's Department of Health and Environmental Control combines public health functions with those of environmental protection. The main public health agency in Maryland is the Department of Health and Mental Hygiene, while in West Virginia the Department of Health and Human Services is the lead public health agency. The Department of Public Health in Kentucky is part of its Cabinet for Health and Family Services.

In nine Appalachian states, environmental health responsibilities are fragmented further into multiple agencies administering environmental protection programs in addition to a public health agency. In these cases, typically one agency regulates pollution while another manages natural resources. Ohio, for example, has three agencies responsible for environmental health: the Ohio Environmental Protection Agency (Ohio EPA), the Ohio Department of Natural Resources (ODNR), and the Ohio Department of Health (ODH). In the ODH's Bureau of Environmental Health there are numerous programs addressing public health issues, including lead abatement, food safety, and public swimming pools. The bureau holds primary responsibility for licensing and certifying professionals and facilities, setting minimum standards to protect public health, and providing technical assistance and training. Even though the ODH has some regulatory responsibility, the local health departments are the crucial link between its mandated programs and the public.

The Ohio EPA enforces federal and state environmental laws and regulates polluters. Its programs include air pollution control, solid and hazardous waste management, emergency response, and water pollution control. Even though the Ohio EPA is the lead regulatory agency, its jurisdiction is focused on public, rather than private, infrastructure. For example, Ohio EPA is responsible for ensuring that publicly owned wastewater and drinking-water treatment plants comply with state and federal laws. On the other hand, local health departments work with the Ohio Department of Health to enforce regulations on private systems, including septic systems and private drinking-water wells.

Historically, programs at ODNR have focused on conservation services, such as providing hunting and fishing licenses, enforcing boating regulations, and managing state parks and natural areas. However, in the context of Appalachian public health issues, ODNR is the lead agency in managing the state's mineral and energy resources, including natural gas extraction from hydraulic fracturing. In a somewhat unusual move, the state legislature gave ODNR the responsibility to monitor potential public health impacts from hydraulic fracturing. It is unusual because Ohio EPA has jurisdiction over enforcing the federal Clean Water Act and Safe Drinking Water Act, two key laws that govern water quality in the state.

The example of the environmental health regulatory scheme in Ohio is one of several that demonstrate challenges in public health protection on the state level. Much like the federal structure, there are multiple agencies influencing environmental health, leading to fragmented state systems with often-confusing overlap. Food safety is a fundamental component of environmental health and there is a disjointed approach in several states due to the existence of multiple programs in different agencies. One agency might oversee food sold directly to consumers, another might inspect food processing facilities, and still another might be responsible for ensuring food safety on farms. In some cases states do not get adequate resources from the federal government for implementing laws, a situation known as unfunded mandates. "No money, no mandate" was part of the battle cry of the US House of Representatives in 1995 when, under Newt Gingrich's leadership, it attempted to roll back regulations, especially those for environmental protection.

In 2017, unfunded mandates surfaced again as part of the argument for easing federal oversight of environmental programs. To some, it seems logical that states should be given resources to implement and enforce federal laws, but this is rarely the case. The most important environmentally related legislation debated and voted on in Washington, DC, is the budget, not any one specific environmental law. Congress creates unfunded mandates in its budget bills, making many local environmental and public health programs ineffective at best and nonexistent at worst. Then, after hamstringing state governments, Congress argues that environmental and public health laws are unenforceable and regulations are out of control. The political and economic conditions within states lead to demands for either more resources or less regulation, and set up conditions for disputes between levels of government.[20]

Disputes between state and federal governments often involve specific issues. Whether it is about expanding Medicaid, supporting same-sex marriage, or legalizing marijuana, state legislatures will take on the federal government, especially when they believe the state's economy is at stake. For example, in many Appalachian places people believe that coal is the answer to their economic woes, including unemployment and poverty. In these places elected officials and residents are hostile to the EPA because they perceive that it is solely responsible for shutting down the coal industry in an overzealous attempt to protect the environment. Driving through Appalachia, you can see evidence of this perception in pro-coal, antigovernment messages on billboards in Pennsylvania and protests over new mining regulations in West Virginia.

In some Appalachian communities, every new federal initiative to control greenhouse gas emissions or focus on greater mine safety is seen as part of the war on coal. This is portrayed as a war because of the passionate belief that the industry is under assault by the federal government and sophisticated environmental activist organizations. Never mind that coal creates environmental mayhem and vast public health maladies. For decades it has been a main source of good jobs, with benefits, throughout Appalachia. Also overlooked is the impact of cheaper natural gas on coal mining as politicians pander to coal interests by joining the front lines in the war with their battle cry of easing regulations. Coal has national environmental, economic, and health implications, but it directly affects the environment, economy, and health of local places throughout Appalachia.

Whether we realize it or not, from the inspector in our neighborhood to the surgeon general in Washington, DC, environmental health professionals are some of the most important public health personnel. Numerous credentials and educational requirements contribute to the breadth and credibility of environmental health practice. The most common credential is Registered Sanitarian/ Registered Environmental Health Specialist (RS/REHS). The RS/REHS is like many other health professions, such as Registered Nurse or Registered Dietician, in terms of educational standards, the need to pass a comprehensive examination, and a required number of annual continuing education credits. Minimum educational standards as set by the National Environmental Health Science and Protection Accreditation Council (EHAC) include basic and organic chemistry, physics, biological sciences, epidemiology, toxicology, and numerous environmental health courses on topics such as food safety, vector control, occupational health, industrial hygiene, and water and air pollution control. At many universities, students who earn a Bachelor of Science degree in Environmental Health complete a curriculum similar to those heading into a career in medicine.

Environmental health practitioners can seek additional certifications and registrations for several specialties, including food safety, lead abatement, solid and hazardous waste, occupational safety, and the built environment. State credentials for environmental health practice are usually coordinated by a board that oversees requirements and sets minimum standards to achieve and maintain registration. The profession is enhanced by specific associations, such as the Georgia Environmental Health Association, or one that covers public health in general, such as the New York State Public Health Association. These organizations are important because they offer professional development opportunities through meetings, trainings, and other types of events. The state registration boards differ from the professional associations because they usually operate under legislation to administer regulations pertaining to credentialing. Credentials are important indicators of a qualified environmental health workforce, but it is up to each state to set minimum qualifications. Many Appalachian states do not require environmental health professionals to attain professional registration to work in the field, an approach that is said by some to be justified by resource conditions in local health agencies.[21]

Local Environmental Health

Just like politics, public health is local. While state governors wrangle with Congress, the White House, and multiple federal agencies over bigger-picture policy and legislative issues, local environmental health professionals still must go about their daily work to protect public health. Housed mainly in state agencies and county and city health departments, these professionals are the frontline personnel for preventing widespread illness and injury. Environmental health practitioners conduct thousands of inspections every year in restaurants, groceries, tattoo parlors, nursing homes, schools, landfills, water treatment facilities, mobile home parks, swimming pools . . . and the list goes on. When not inspecting facilities for compliance with regulations, they are responding to complaints and concerns about mosquitoes, rats, rabies, litter, noise, smells, and many other matters. They affect everyone every day.

Without local environmental health professionals, public health in the United States would collapse. The foundation has been cracking for years because most local health agencies rely on limited and uncertain funding to accomplish their missions. Prevention is perceived as expensive and, with competing demands for diminishing local resources, health agencies are often underfunded and desperately shorthanded. Even in states on sound financial footing, public health programs are seldom prioritized over economic growth, so the situation in the thirteen states comprising Appalachia is even more critical.

Conditions are especially dire in localities that rely on state and local taxes to support their work, a circumstance that underscores the direct relationship between poverty and environmental health. Counties with high poverty and unemployment will have fewer tax resources dedicated to health priorities because of the competition from education, economic development, public safety, and other social services. This competition is intensified because Appalachian counties are among the poorest counties in their respective states, a fact that directly affects local environmental health.

The local environmental health infrastructure in Appalachian states varies from regional, multicounty approaches to those delineated by county or city boundaries. Alabama employs a regional approach to environmental health and delineates eleven public health areas with a local health officer in each area. Nine of the eleven areas include multiple counties; two of the areas consist of one county: Jefferson County, home of Birmingham, and Mobile County, home of Mobile. The sixty-five counties that comprise the nine multiple-county health areas are supported with state funds only. Within each county there are also local health departments to provide clinical services, home health care, medical social work, and environmental services pertaining to food service, hotels, jails, body art facilities, onsite wastewater systems, solid waste management facilities and transportation, rabies and vector control, public health nuisances, and private drinking water. Alabama's system is like those of other Appalachian states in its reliance on local agencies as the key inspection and enforcement bodies for many important programs. However, Alabama is somewhat unique because these local agencies do not rely on local taxes as much as in some of the other states in the region.

In contrast to Alabama, there are more than a hundred local health departments in Ohio, some of which serve only cities while others combine city and county or are single-county health districts. In addition, some cities contract with local health departments to meet their environmental health mandates. The local health departments have their own governing bodies in boards of health, and they count on local taxpayers to support their programs through levies and local government budgets. This means that the finances of local health departments mirror those of school districts in Ohio and require political and public support. Residents must routinely vote to increase or maintain their local taxes to support public services, so local health departments may struggle to meet their mandates, let alone offer additional programs to improve public health.

Dependence on local health departments for environmental health inspections and enforcement activity is not unique to Appalachia. Nationwide, environmental health practice is variously constrained by inadequacy of resources, including personnel and money, by the geographic range of local environmental specialists, and/or by an absence of requirements for credentialed professionals. In the face of most of such constraints, local governments in Appalachia lack the ability to adequately implement environmental health programs because of the pressing needs of programs not focused on the environment. Environmental health is just one public health component among many in local health agencies. Others include vaccination, food and nutrition (including WIC and SNAP programs), health education, and numerous health and safety programs such as those providing and certifying car seats or encouraging smoking cessation. As obesity and diabetes, smoking, and opioid addiction have become public health priorities in Appalachia, safeguarding adequate resources for routine environmental health activities such as restaurant inspections and mosquito surveillance remains a challenge.

SHIFTING THE HEALTH PARADIGM

Protecting public health through environmental health programs involves a multitude of players at all levels of government, from global initiatives in the hands of international organizations to local sanitarians inspecting restaurants. Globally, many organizations prioritize projects to reduce health disparities that are associated with environmental health inequities. International declarations drawing attention to social determinants of health and global programs linking environmental exposures to health outcomes have not filtered down to people who live in rural Appalachia. Until there is a paradigm shift toward recognizing the importance of environmental and public health in the United States, including the inequities that exist in specific places as well as in public health programs and policies, health disparities will persist.

Shifting the US health paradigm to one of prevention rather than treatment will take both education and political resolve. Individual access to preventive healthcare can be expensive, but preventive public health programs are often less so. Recent evidence related to public health spending paints a bleak picture of the potential for its success. Budgets for federal public health agencies continually suffer staggering cuts as national priorities remain focused on insuring individuals rather than protecting public health.[22] Public health budgets at the state and local levels have suffered even greater losses as most states have decreased their budgets and per capita spending has been cut dramatically.

Health inequities are preventable, and robust environmental health programs are a critical component of prevention. The elaborate environmental health infrastructure existing at all governmental levels creates opportunities and challenges for addressing place-based exposures that contribute to these inequities. The challenges include funding currently being tied to wealth and the need to carefully administer scarce resources. Opportunities also exist for local environmental exposures to be managed by those most directly affected. As the stories in the following chapters suggest, there are environmental exposures that are unique or intensified in Appalachia, and preventing these exposures will likely remain a significant focus of environmental health in these places for years to come.

2

A Place for the Built Environment and Health

> While there are services available to the poor in Appalachia, the rural nature of the area and the remoteness of local communities make it difficult for these services to be delivered, especially in times of emergency. These are the people in the greatest need of health care, yet the rural nature of the area makes it hard to sustain a physician in a remote community. Plus, transportation services are not provided to cover rural areas and many poor residents do not own vehicles to travel to doctors and hospitals in larger cities well over an hour away. Thus, many Appalachia residents are in serious jeopardy from what are usually routine health problems in rural areas.
>
> —Appalachian environmental health professional

FOREST COUNTY IN WESTERN PENNSYLVANIA IS A COMPELLING case study of the built environment in Appalachia. In 2000, 4,946 people lived in Forest County; by 2010 the county's population had grown to 7,716 people. More interesting than the overall population growth is the fact that the male population almost doubled, from 2,604 in 2000 to 5,164 in 2010, while the female population only grew by 210. Also interesting is that this county in the heart of rural western Pennsylvania includes 1,389 black males, almost 18 percent of the county's population. Does this population growth signify a major industry opening in the county? Does it mean that the county is on the road to economic recovery after decades of decline? When we investigate the underlying reason for the demographic shift in the county, the growth is not related to improving economic conditions, even though local politicians have advertised it as such. In fact, Forest County was ranked as one of the fastest-growing counties between 2000 and 2010 because of a new prison. The state correctional institution (SCI Forest) opened in 2004 and as of October 2019 housed 2,152 male offenders in a facility designed for 2,306.[1]

The prison scenario in Forest County is familiar in Appalachia, where local politicians often promote controversial developments as solutions to economic woes to gain public support. Officials exaggerate estimates for new jobs linked to these projects and local people often do not benefit from the hype. In the case of SCI Forest, local elected officials courted the facility's developers because they believed it would promote economic development in the county. According to the Pennsylvania Department of Corrections, when they were looking for a place to build a new state prison, their search "caught the attention of Forest County Commissioners." A major employer in the county had recently closed and "the Commissioners decided a state-run corrections facility would be a boost to the area."[2]

County officials worked diligently to get the prison built, and the first inmates began arriving in October 2004. SCI Forest provides full-time jobs for more than 650 people, but not all these employees are local residents. Meanwhile, Forest County has some of the highest poverty and unemployment rates in the state, including a percentage of children who live in poverty that is twice the state average. Forest County is the only county in Pennsylvania that the Appalachian Regional Commission rated "distressed" in 2020, meaning that it is one of the most economically distressed counties in the country.

When it comes to health, the Robert Wood Johnson Foundation's 2019 County Health Rankings also paint a gloomy picture of Forest County.[3] Of the sixty-seven counties in Pennsylvania, Forest County ranks sixty-fifth in terms of health factors such as smoking, obesity, access to food, excessive drinking, and teen births. Additionally, the county ranks low for access to clinical care and multiple social and economic factors. To put this in perspective, according to many indicators the urban Philadelphia County is the only other county in the state that ranks lower for many health factors. Forest County suffers from a lack of primary care doctors, dentists, and mental health providers. Researchers trying to understand health disparities between poor people and those more well-off often focus indicators such as health care access, lifestyle choices, and inadequate insurance. While these factors clearly contribute to health disparities, many differences in health status can at least be partially explained by living conditions, or the built environment.

The built environment includes inside and outside spaces. Both affect health in positive and negative ways. Homes, schools, hospitals, day care centers, parks, and entire neighborhoods are components of the built environment. A health-conscious built environment involves more than just maintaining adequate distances from environmental risks, it incorporates how communities are designed and planned as well as housing and institutional conditions. The built environment contributes to health disparities that are intimately tied to place and we must look past broad environmental indicators such as air and water quality to fully understand its health impacts. This is especially important in Appalachia because the environmental splendor can camouflage how place affects health. Residents of Forest County live in one of the most beautiful places in Pennsylvania, but they are also in one of the unhealthiest places in the state. While decision makers focused their attention on building a prison, the built environment in the rest of the county continued to decline.

In Forest County, the air is relatively clean and drinking water is relatively safe for those who are on public systems. Upon closer examination, however, you can find underlying environmental issues surfacing related to housing. Almost 75 percent of homes in the county are identified in the census as "vacant." This alarmingly high percentage of vacant housing is due to "seasonal, recreational, or occasional use" homes: Forest County is a major vacation spot for hunting, fishing, and enjoying nature. However, what has been historically a seasonal phenomenon is evolving into something more permanent as vacation homes are being converted to year-round housing. Most of these homes were built on small lots during a time of more lax water and sewer regulations, so the safety of the county's drinking water and the ability to manage wastewater are becoming critical environmental health issues. As the county's community development plan puts it, "Remote concentrations of seasonal-use properties that are interspersed with year-round residences are creating and exasperating issues with failing on-lot septic systems."[4]

While environmental health problems intensify for Forest County residents, the state of Pennsylvania has spent millions maintaining and upgrading the prison. In 2013, the Department of Corrections spent $4 million replacing the hot water piping distribution system in the facility. This was followed a year later by $1.4 million to replace the security fencing. These projects pale in comparison to the $17.5 million for the 2012 construction project allowing the facility to include 128 new beds.[5] Overall, the Department of Corrections estimated that it cost $38,331 for each inmate at SCI Forest in 2016.[6] Meanwhile, the median household income in Forest County from 2013 through 2017 was $37,106.[7]

There are sixty-seven counties in Pennsylvania and only six county and four municipal health departments. Public health in many rural areas falls under the jurisdiction of the state Department of Health. There is no local health department in Forest County, so those making decisions about the built environment are detached from those responsible for public health. There are two local planning units in Forest County government: the Conservation District and Planning Department and the Community and Economic Development Department. The Conservation District and Planning Department Board prepared the county's comprehensive plan, which prioritizes improving infrastructure with minimal attention to public health. The Community Development Plan from the Community and Economic Development Department also focuses on infrastructure improvements, noting that "infrastructure issues are one of the most serious problems plaguing Forest County."[8] Even though both plans mention public health, promoting economic development while conserving the rural character of the county are the main motivations for strategies.

Almost ten years after the prison opened, local officials engaged in a planning process focused on the future of the county. Their 2013 county comprehensive plan notes that "prisoners do not contribute directly to the local economy, and pay no local taxes. The Prison may very well cost the County more than it benefits it."[9] While the prison was being built, the county upgraded a sewage treatment plant to handle the wastewater from the influx of several thousand prisoners. New infrastructure was also installed to provide the prison access to a public water system. You can see these improvements as you drive toward the prison along the heavily forested road. The fire hydrants stop right after the prison. So, among the recent environmental health improvements in the county, many have directly benefited prisoners rather than residents, and county planners are still focused on the goal of providing "adequate clean and healthy water resources" to all residents of the county.[10]

Infrastructure is the backbone of places that grow and thrive. It is also one cornerstone of healthy built environments. Roads, water supplies, sewers, cell phone and internet services, and waste management benefit residents and can improve local environmental conditions. When places such as Forest County engage in comprehensive planning, they tend to focus on improving transportation networks, expanding water services, and augmenting public infrastructure as keys to enhancing their communities. More recently, planners and public health professionals see parks, street trees, bike lanes, and other recreational areas as critical elements of healthy communities. While this connection to community planning may seem like a new approach to public health, it defined the profession more than 150 years ago.

PLANNING, PUBLIC HEALTH, AND THE BUILT ENVIRONMENT

In the middle of a steamy August in 1858, the city of London was "brought to its knees" because of the disgusting odor of the Thames River.[11] For decades, people used the river as a receptacle for all kinds of waste, including dead animals, human sewage, and commercial rubbish, but the city ignored the problem until the heat cooked up the smell. Parliament closed and the public demanded that something be done to clean up what was considered the dirtiest river in the world. How the city dealt with the "Great Stink" is an example of an infrastructure project that set the stage for including public health in planning decisions and led to the sanitary reform movement. The goal of the movement was to minimize the "filth" considered the source of disease and illness.[12] Sanitary reformers went to work devising ways to separate people from obvious environmental insults. They designed and installed systems to move dirty water away from cities and clean drinking water into cities. Those planning water transport and treatment systems in the late 1800s were early public health practitioners. Even though their main goal was to abate nuisances, they directly promoted health.

The installation of water infrastructure more than a hundred years ago demonstrates the relationship between the built environment and health, and that thoughtful planning can minimize exposures to environmental hazards. Since the Great Stink, both the planning and public health professions have evolved, and not all the evolution has been good for creating healthy places. In fact, some of least healthy places are the result of policy decisions to specifically disconnect planning and public health. Today, state and local governments in the United States typically separate departments of planning and public health, a situation that leads to competition for scarce resources. This situation also contributes to trade-offs between economic development and public and environmental health in local decision making.

The American Public Health Association (APHA) defines healthy communities as those that meet the basic needs of every individual and provide "quality and sustainability of the environment through tobacco and smoke-free spaces, clean air, soil and water, green and open spaces, and sustainable energy use."[13] The APHA, the CDC, and the US Public Health Service are calling attention to the role of place, particularly the built environment, in public health. They are investigating the impacts of social, economic, and environmental influences on chronic community health issues such as obesity. By paying attention to the built environment, place has become a key focus of public health.

Understanding and addressing the relationship between the built environment and health requires a renewed commitment to city and regional planning and to rebuilding the tenuous relationship between public health practitioners and city and regional planners. Suburban neighborhoods are a perfect example of this relationship. If planners and developers of these sprawling, automobile-dependent neighborhoods considered public health impacts, perhaps we would have less of them. Cul-de-sacs, garages as one of the most significant features of every home, and the lack of community amenities within walkable distances from residences rob daily life of physical activity. In retrospect, many believe this type of neighborhood design has contributed to the obesity epidemic.

It has taken some time, but influential agencies and organizations are revisiting historic neighborhood-design elements that encourage walking and cycling for transportation. For example, the CDC's Healthy Community Design Initiative focuses on improving public health by encouraging community planners to include health in all the planning decisions made at the local level.[14] Like politics and public health, most planning is local, so community residents and their elected officials can have a significant voice in creating healthy built environments. The goals of the federal government's Healthy People 2020 initiative support healthy communities and homes with specific objectives for improving indoor air quality, mitigating exposure to lead-based products, and reducing poor housing quality.[15] All of this comes down to the role of place in creating, maintaining, or intensifying circumstances that make some people less healthy than others.

Leading public health organizations at all levels of government are now seeking to answer the question, How important is your zip code to your health? Like environmental justice research, much of the healthy places discourse has occurred in urban studies. We have not paid enough attention to the impact of place on health in rural communities. This is one reason why facilities such as the prison in Forest County garner support from local officials. Poor communication between departments of planning and public health can lead local officials to implement development strategies without considering their potentially harmful environmental and health impacts. This is especially problematic in areas that are economically distressed. For decades, an approach encouraging economic development at all costs has been prominent throughout Appalachia because of unemployment and poverty concerns. When planners emphasize projects to improve the economy, they can create both negative and positive health outcomes.

In some instances, infrastructure projects in Appalachia provide greater economic benefits to those outside of the region than those within it. Boosting the region's economy is the overarching goal for enhancing transportation infrastructure in Appalachia. The Appalachian Regional Commission's main mission for more than fifty years has been to improve transportation in the region. Specifically, one of the four goals of the Commission is implementing the Appalachian Development Highway System (ADHS). The rationale for emphasizing transportation infrastructure is to benefit the local and regional economies by connecting places in Appalachia to the rest of the country. The ADHS includes plans for more than three thousand miles of highways, more than 90 percent of which have already been completed.[16] Many of the roads in the ADHS are high-speed highways and, in many cases, these roads bypass local communities. As a result, people and products can get through Appalachia quickly without slowing down to support local businesses.

Building new roads certainly makes travel more efficient, but there are other consequences that may not be as obvious. Well-planned transportation systems can make physical activity easier or more difficult, reduce or exacerbate air pollution, and increase or decrease death, mental health, and stress. Transportation planning that emphasizes improving conditions for cars rather than people can influence inequities and enhance health disparities. Car-focused planning rarely considers public health implications. In the legislative and planning documents for the ADHS there is no indication that public health was discussed in crafting the transportation strategy for Appalachia. These documents do not mention the residual public health impacts created when rural people are suddenly surrounded by a high-speed highway. Nor is there any mention of how rerouting thousands of people around local businesses may actually lead to less healthy communities because of the loss of revenues that form the foundation for public health programs.

Improving transportation efficiency by building new roads creates a public health paradox in that it can improve access to health care while at the same time increase the risk of negative health outcomes. In order to have the most positive influence on public health, transportation planners should focus on increasing mobility through multimodal approaches that include promoting and designing places with pedestrians, rather than cars, in mind. Of course, these types of approaches work well in urban areas, but they may not apply in rural Appalachia. Nevertheless, an emerging planning approach, the Health Impact Assessment (HIA), shows some promise in integrating planning and public health for major policy decisions affecting the built environment.

The HIA is similar to federally mandated Environmental Impact Assessments (EIAs), which are required for all significant development projects using federal funding. The Appalachian Development Highway System is an example of an endeavor requiring an EIA. The EIA looks at environmental impacts such as wildlife habitat fragmentation, detriment to water quality, and loss of endangered species. Public health has never been a component of EIAs and, until recently, evaluating potential health impacts has been left out of land-use planning. HIAs are still voluntary, but their use is growing as a tool to ensure healthy places and address the root causes of poor health. Through its Built Environment and Health Initiative, the CDC is advocating the use of HIAs in transportation planning and other major development projects and policy decisions.[17]

An HIA involves multiple steps and requires community members to be engaged throughout the process. Numerous successful projects have demonstrated how an HIA can accomplish development goals and minimize health impacts.[18] Because an HIA involves community members and public health professionals in forecasting a range of health outcomes from built environment programs and policies, it includes alternatives to ensure public health is maintained or even advanced with each new project. There is no mandate for HIAs, so planners and developers are not required to proactively assess potential health effects of most major development projects, including the prison in Forest County, Pennsylvania, or the high-speed highways cutting through Appalachia. These types of projects are only one component of how the built environment affects healthy places at a macro level. There are also microlevel conditions in the built environment that contribute to the health status of people who live in Appalachia.

One consequence of poverty is that poor people live, work, and play in places that lack adequate infrastructure and other services and sometimes are simply unhealthy. While officials plan prisons and major highway construction projects using extensive government resources, the conditions of inside places are left in the hands of local people. These conditions are related to an array of environmental health issues. Diseases spread by vectors such as fleas, cockroaches, and rodents thrive in places where sanitation is weakest. Housing and other inside places in areas poorly drained due to inadequate maintenance or shoddy construction are havens for mosquitoes to spread disease. Neglected housing stock encourages high mold levels, leading to health conditions such as allergies and asthma. Inside many homes and schools, children are exposed to deteriorating lead paint and secondhand smoke, underscoring the impact of the micro-level built environment on cognition and development.

Indoor environments can be as toxic as outside environments. Pollution can be more concentrated inside places and exposures are longer due to the amount of time people spend inside. The EPA identifies indoor air quality as an environmental justice issue because low-income people and minorities are not only more likely to be exposed to many indoor toxins, but are also less likely to have the resources to mitigate these exposures.[19] Many of the environmental health concerns associated with inside places are not unique to Appalachia. However, in some cases, there is a greater potential for exposure in Appalachia based on geology, geography, and ecology. The health impacts from inside environments intensify when exposures to specific risks combine with other inequities. Radon is one of these specific risks and could be one of the most important built environment concerns in Appalachia.

Radon

Radon is perhaps the most significant and least understood environmental health problem. Radon is a naturally occurring radioactive gas emitted from uranium, so its levels are place-specific and linked to local geology. Unlike wave radiation, such as ultraviolet radiation from the sun, which is absorbed through the skin, radon is particle radiation and can be inhaled or ingested. Because radon comes from rock underlying built places, radon levels are typically highest in basements. Radioactive particles can enter structures through cracks in foundations, gaps around plumbing and ventilation pipes, or pits that contain sump pumps. People who live in areas with high levels of radon can inhale the airborne particles while sitting in their basements, taking a shower, or drinking well water. Over time, the radiation accumulates in the lungs and contributes to the risk of lung cancer. Many health experts believe that radon is a leading cause of lung cancer, second only to cigarette smoke.[20]

Radon is relatively easy to abate and generally just requires improving ventilation to release it to the outside air. However, to alleviate radon, you must know it exists. Not many people are even aware of the risks from radon exposure, let alone how much radon is in their homes. The EPA and other federal agencies are so concerned about low levels of testing that they created a National Radon Action Plan with the goal of saving thirty-two hundred lives by the year 2020.[21] This plan is a partnership between multiple governmental agencies and nonprofits and builds from previous initiatives to educate the public about radon risks, support testing, and mitigate the risks in millions of homes, schools, and other facilities. A key strategy for reducing radon risk is to integrate radon reduction materials and design into the housing sector. Other strategies include requiring disclosure of radon levels during real estate transactions, strengthening local building codes, and developing a source of funds for low-income people to test for and mitigate radon in places where people cannot afford to do this without financial support. The EPA did create a radon grant program for state governments to apply for funds to offset costs of their own programs, but hardly any of the 2015 Radon Action Plan has been implemented.

Lung cancer mortality rates are significantly higher in Appalachia than in the rest of the country.[22] This may not be surprising considering the high smoking rates in the region. The combined effects of smoking, poverty, and educational attainment are not the only risk factors for developing lung cancer; we must also consider geology. It is possible that radon plays a role in cancer incidence in Appalachia, especially considering that "radon is the number one cause of lung cancer among nonsmokers."[23] Consider the evidence that living in the coalfields of Appalachia correlates with high levels of lung cancer.[24] Mining, processing, and burning coal create air pollutants such as arsenic and fine particles that carry toxins deep into the lungs and many common coal-related pollutants are associated with lung cancers. Radon is a lesser-known environmental health risk from coal, but some studies confirm that levels of radon inside coal mines could be endangering the health of workers in these mines.[25] Radiation is released when coal is burned to generate electricity, but airborne radiation in the outside environment might not be the greatest risk of radiation exposure in the coalfields. Proximity to coal may be an important indicator of potential for exposure to radon regardless of where the power plant is located.

The risk of being exposed to indoor radon is a function of the integrity of building foundations and local geology. Everyone is exposed to some level of radon, but there are some places where exposures are greater than others. The EPA categorizes areas of the United States as being part of one of three zones based on high, moderate, or low potential radon exposure.[26] These zones are delineated by geology, soil structure, some indoor measurements, and radio-activity as measured in the air. The zones are not identified as the result of wide-spread testing for radon in buildings, but on indicators that might contribute to indoor levels. Overall, the EPA identifies the upper Midwest, some portions of the Southwest, and along the Appalachian Mountains as places with the greatest potential for exposure. Within the thirteen states in the region, areas with the highest potential for radon exposure are concentrated in those counties demarcated as Appalachian by the Appalachian Regional Commission. This is also where the coal is.

Deteriorating building conditions exacerbate exposure to radon. Older homes with cracked foundations and poor ventilation are prime environments for high levels of indoor radon. Households using private well water are also at risk of exposure because their water is not monitored for radon as it would be with a public drinking-water system. Geology, housing stock, and source of water combine to underscore the need for examining the impact of radon on lung cancer rates in Appalachia, especially in rural areas bordering the mountains and communities near coal mining sites. Nevertheless, one of the main problems with understanding the health impacts of radon in Appalachia is that, while it is a credible threat, it is not one that can be accurately assessed without testing. Considering that radon is a leading cause of lung cancer, that lung cancer rates are higher in Appalachian counties than others, and that geological conditions in the region enhance exposure to radon, targeting resources to address this problem should be an important public health priority.

Most public health departments do not monitor radon exposures because there are no mandates and resources to do so. Instead, radon is mostly managed via educational programs encouraging residents to test their homes using free test kits. For example, West Virginia's 2016–20 Cancer Plan includes one general aim (out of twenty-five) targeting non-tobacco-related environmental exposures. The specific objectives include increasing "radon test kits provided to the public each year from 999 to 1,500" and educating "the public annually on environmental and/or occupational carcinogens."[27] Without financial support, regulatory mandates, and public outrage, radon exposures will continue unabated, and we will never get a sense of the magnitude of this serious public health problem in Appalachia. It may be time to apply lessons learned from managing exposures to other contaminants, such as lead, which is a somewhat successful case study of a place-based environmental health threat.

Lead

As with radon, housing conditions contribute to lead exposure. Like radon, lead occurs naturally in the environment, but it is a heavy metal rather than a radioactive element. Health effects from exposure to high levels of many heavy metals are well known and similar. We know that these substances can accumulate in the body and cause neurological problems. We also know that there are multiple exposure routes, some of which we can control and others we cannot. Much of our exposure to lead has not been because it occurs naturally in water, like arsenic, or because it is emitted into the air as a by-product of burning coal, like mercury. Rather, we have created extensive exposures by adding lead to products such as gasoline and paint to improve their performance. So, while the health effects of lead are like those from other heavy metals, the circumstances leading to so many people being affected are similar to chemicals like asbestos. Older houses are saturated with lead and asbestos because they cheaply enhanced construction materials.

We have been exposed to lead by drinking water flowing through lead-soldered plumbing, ingesting lead dust from paint, or breathing emissions from cars running on leaded gasoline. If public health professionals had never linked lead to developmental delays in children, that contact with lead might have continued. Reducing lead exposure is one of the great public health success stories in the United States, starting with the removal of lead from gasoline. Congress passed legislation mandating a phase-out of lead as a constituent of gasoline beginning in 1973, with total elimination by 1995. This legislation and the regulatory action that followed resulted in a tremendous decrease in lead measured in the outside environment and in the number of children with high levels of lead in their blood.

The CDC started collecting data on blood lead levels in 1997 through the National Health and Nutrition Examination Survey (NHANES). This survey began in the 1960s to assess the health of Americans and is regularly revised to include new public health concerns as they emerge. NHANES includes data from questionnaires as well as physical examinations and laboratory test results. According to the survey, lead levels in American children have been decreasing since 1999.[28] This indicates a major improvement in public health, and much of the success is attributable to banning lead in gasoline and minimizing its use in consumer products, including paint.

Reducing health impacts from lead has been successful but NHANES data suggest some disproportionate exposures to be concerned about. For example, survey results clearly indicate a higher percentage of elevated blood lead levels in children who live in homes built before 1950. These older homes were built at a time when lead paint was ubiquitous. In addition, children who live in poverty and are enrolled in Medicaid have higher lead levels than those who are not poor and not served by Medicaid. So, while the country has benefited overall from eliminating lead in gasoline, childhood lead poisoning is now an environmental justice issue disproportionately affecting poor children who live in older homes.

Once lead was phased out of gasoline, it became more of an environmental health concern in inside places. Structures built before the ban may still have high amounts of lead-based paint and children living in these homes are suffering the consequences. According to the US census, about 18 percent of homes in the United States and 22 percent of those in the Appalachian states were built before 1950. Almost half of the homes within the thirteen Appalachian states were built before 1970. It is not surprising that New York and Pennsylvania have the oldest housing stock in the region because these figures include the entire state, so they are influenced by major cities such as Philadelphia and New York. Investigating inequitable exposures to lead in rural areas is challenging because public health professionals must rely on local health statistics that are incomplete and often unavailable.

In the absence of reliable local statistics, we must turn to national and state-wide surveys to observe lead exposures. Through the NHANES the CDC compiles blood lead levels and reports state-level data. There are significant limitations with blood lead data that make it difficult to compare places. These limitations include different testing methods, rationale for testing children, and the absence of coordinated approaches to lead testing. Up to 2012, the CDC used 10 micrograms of lead per deciliter of whole blood as the level of concern; if children tested at this level or above, action to eliminate exposure was encouraged or required in some instances. In 2012, CDC reviewed the science behind lead health effects and reduced the action level to 5 micrograms based on the opinion that no exposure to lead is safe.

CDC data indicate the highest percentage of children with elevated lead levels live in Pennsylvania. However, this is not unequivocal, due to the measurement limitations.[29] Laboratory data from Pennsylvania indicate that a little more than 3 percent of the children tested had elevated blood lead levels in 2017.[30] It may be comforting to see such low percentages of children with high blood lead levels, but keep in mind that only a small percentage of children are tested. Expanding testing to include more children, especially those in rural areas, could either increase or decrease the magnitude of the problem. Until resources exist to broaden testing efforts, we will have to estimate and extrapolate in order to understand the burden of lead in Appalachia.[31]

Forty-eight of Pennsylvania's sixty-seven counties are considered rural according to the definition used by the Center for Rural Pennsylvania. This definition is based on population density as measured by the 2010 United States Census, and all counties with less than 284 people per square mile are identified as rural.[32] All but one of the rural counties in Pennsylvania are located within the Appalachian region of the state and about 25 percent of the state's children under the age of seven live in these counties. Although the counties encompassing and surrounding Philadelphia have high percentages of homes built before 1978, the counties comprising the Appalachian portion of the state have higher percentages of older housing stock than those not in the region. This means that housing in rural Pennsylvania likely contributes to unmeasured childhood lead exposure in the state.

It is worth repeating that we must interpret blood lead levels measured in rural Appalachia with caution. Since kids in rural Appalachian counties are less likely to be tested than those in the more urban areas, relying on national or statewide testing could misrepresent the magnitude of childhood lead poisoning. If estimates concerning the inadequate coverage of lead testing in rural areas are accurate, it is almost certain that many children in Appalachia are not being tested or treated for lead-related conditions. In addition, since local health departments are often tasked with monitoring and responding to high lead levels, local resources certainly play a role in addressing this important public health problem.

Regardless of testing protocols and practices, lead poisoning in children remains an important public health concern. Decades of research identifies cognitive, behavioral, and neurological effects from lead exposure. Because lead accumulates in the body, lead poisoning can result in long-term health effects, inhibiting development and a child's ability to learn. Furthermore, studies have linked prenatal exposures and high blood lead levels to attention deficit hyperactivity disorder (ADHD) in children.[33] ADHD is an increasingly common concern, especially since it can lead to long-term consequences, including substance abuse, which is one of the most important public health challenges in Appalachia.

Secondhand Smoke

Some research has also linked prenatal exposure to cigarette smoke with ADHD, although conclusions about this relationship are more uncertain. Regardless of the connection to ADHD, children are at risk from exposure to secondhand tobacco smoke. While smoking rates have declined in the United States since 1960, rates in Appalachia remain higher than in other regions of the country. Health effects of smoking are well known. They include cancer, heart disease, and chronic obstructive pulmonary disease (COPD), among many others. Smoking is a problem in Appalachia, especially in Kentucky, which has the highest percentage of smokers in the country. Kentucky also has the highest cancer rates in the country, with eastern and southeastern Appalachian counties leading the way.[34] Kentucky's prevalence rate for lung cancer is almost double the national rate.[35]

The seeds of the public health consequences of smoking were planted in Kentucky a long time ago. Kentucky has high rates of lung cancer, high rates of smokers, and it is a place where a lot of tobacco is grown. Kentucky and North Carolina grow most of the tobacco in the United States.[36] Although tobacco farming is declining, it is still a major contributor to the agricultural economy in these states.[37] Much like the prison case in Forest County built with local support because of perceived economic benefits, support for tobacco is also tied to the economies of specific places.

Being diagnosed with lung cancer from smoking is a weighty health issue, but being diagnosed with lung cancer as an innocent bystander while someone else smokes is even more tragic. Secondhand or passive smoking is part of the public health effects from smoking because of the proven connections to cardiovascular disease, cancers, and even sudden infant death syndrome.[38] Living in Appalachia is a significant risk factor for exposure to secondhand smoke, and as with radon and lead exposure, children living in rural Appalachia may be the most vulnerable group in the region.[39]

The disparity of state and local laws regulating smoking inside places where people live, work, and play contributes to inequities in exposure to secondhand smoke. Appalachian states have generally been slower than others to pass statewide smoking bans, leaving nonsmokers at risk of health effects.[40] Numerous states in the United States have comprehensive smoking bans that include bars and restaurants. Of the twelve states that do not have comprehensive smoking laws, seven are in the ARC-designated Appalachian region.[41]

Passing smoking bans in tobacco-growing states has proven to be extremely difficult if not impossible. In February 2015, the Kentucky House of Representatives passed a bill that would ban smoking in workplaces and public spaces, but not bars or restaurants. One month later, the bill was labeled "dead" because it could not pass the senate. Because the state has not been successful in establishing policies to ban indoor smoking, some local places are taking matters into their own hands. For example, the Appalachian Regional Commission identifies McCreary County, Kentucky as a "bright spot" because it was able to implement smoking bans locally.[42]

Curtailing smoking is a public health challenge regardless of the presence of comprehensive smoking laws. This challenge is even greater in the Appalachian region where the absence of laws combines with tobacco's economic role. Education and health promotion can only go so far in addressing smoking prevalence. There are underlying social and economic determinants to address and many of these are out of the hands of public health professionals. Until some of these determinants are attended to, smoking-related diseases will continue to contribute to health disparities in Appalachia. Smoking, like radon and lead, is an environmental health issue tied to inequitable exposures in inside places. The outside places in Appalachia are also sources of environmental health inequities that influence health disparities.

THE BUILT ENVIRONMENT: OUTSIDE PLACES

There is little doubt that community design of the mid-to-late twentieth century contributed to and exacerbated many public health problems. The predominant design strategy of American suburban neighborhoods featured cul-de-sacs, garages as a main housing feature, and backyards with decks and patios instead of front porches. New schools built on large tracts of land instead of near houses meant that the only way kids could get to them was by bus or car. In general, these types of communities were designed for cars, not people, and pedestrians were nothing but a nuisance.

As these neighborhoods popped up around the country, not only did commutes get longer, but the vitality of the central city was jeopardized. After decades of this kind of growth, public health professionals noticed that Americans were gaining weight, especially American children. Then, after gathering data about what is now referred to as the obesity epidemic, experts began to discover that its roots were lodged not only in the way people eat and other health behaviors. They raised questions about how community design and the built environment might contribute to the health-related impacts from obesity.

Food access is discussed elsewhere in this book, but it does relate directly to obesity in the context of the built environment. At least one contributing factor to obesity has to do with the decline of the local grocery store. Those making land-use decisions have not only engineered physical activity out of daily life; they have also inadvertently wiped out accessible local sources of food. There are no longer grocery stores in many communities, especially rural ones. Instead, they are on the fringes of towns, consuming acres of land and requiring people to drive to get to them. Once there, shoppers find that the least healthy foods are the cheapest, so it makes sense to spend their limited dollars on quantity rather than quality. It is a mistake to think that having more farmers' markets and more restaurants using local foods offers a viable, equitable solution. The local-foods movement is not the magic bullet for solving food insecurity that it is advertised to be, because it tends to target the wealthier among us. When it comes to improving access to fresh, healthy foods, land-use planning decisions that pit big-box stores against local groceries are important indicators of this access.

Focusing only on food intake will not solve the obesity epidemic, in any case, because of the challenges involved in using health education or mandates to change eating behaviors. For example, even if school lunches are completely revamped to include only healthy choices, kids will still eat what they like, and what they like may not be the healthiest options. School-age children throw a lot of food away at the end of their lunch period, costing school districts hundreds of thousands of dollars every year. If children are not eating what is served in school and childhood obesity rates continue to rise, then there are clearly other aspects at play.

One thing not at play is the children. Many school districts have removed physical education as part of the regular curriculum to emphasize student testing, and incidental physical activity is not part of the daily lives of large numbers of children. In rural places, children often spend a sizeable amount of time on buses being transported to and from the only school in their county. Once they arrive at school, there is no gym class, and without physical education in the curriculum, many kids have lost their only source of activity. While we may lament the amount of screen time in front of devices, we cannot overlook structural changes in education policy, such as curriculum change and rural school district consolidation, that contribute to one in six children in the United States being obese.

In Appalachia, obesity and its related health problems are endemic, so it is not surprising that diabetes is widespread in the region. The highest rates of diabetes among adults are consistently in Appalachia, with Mississippi and West Virginia often ranking first and second.[43] Searching for the underlying causes of obesity in Appalachia is challenging and researchers are examining demographic factors such as income and education levels.[44] Documenting the built environment impacts on health in Appalachia is difficult because of the physical nature of the region. In many rural areas, children have never had access to sidewalks, bike trails, or parks for physical activity, and walking to school is not an option. As such, health-based community design will take a different form in rural Appalachia and might include small local playgrounds, designated walking paths, and perhaps even organized transportation to access opportunities for group exercise. Planning decisions affect public health in both positive and negative ways, and just paying attention to the health impacts of the built environment is a first step to enhancing the positive impacts.

AILING IN THE BUILT ENVIRONMENT

Many health indicators document that people in rural Appalachia are sicker and feel less healthy than the rest of the country. To understand why this is so, we must look beyond access to medical care and toward underlying place-based factors that contribute to health. We know that designing places with public health in mind can make people healthier without requiring major lifestyle changes. Prioritizing public health is complicated because economic conditions in the poorest Appalachian counties often dictate planning decisions. In these cases, local planners and policymakers promote projects that increase health disparities by enhancing inequitable exposures to unhealthy environmental conditions.

Rural Appalachia does not have many of the built-environment problems of large cities. In these communities you will not see traffic jams and you can find places for solitude and outdoor recreation. However, Appalachia's beauty can mask its underlying health disparities. Historically, those who plan for housing, education, transportation, and tourism have not factored in the health aspects of decisions. Their focus has been on economic consequences of the built environment. It is somewhat of a paradox, then, that in attempting to implement policies to minimize economic disparities, local officials have maximized health disparities.

The good news is that planning and public health are coming together again to address problems created by their historic lack of coordination. For example, the American Planning Association (APA) and the American Public Health Association (APHA) are working together to assist localities in integrating "planning and public health where people live, work and play." Their initiative is called Plan4Health and its mission is to involve local communities in building capacity to improve health, specifically in the domains of nutrition and physical activity. Plan4Health provides funding to local coalitions around the country. However, communities in the Appalachian region are not participating in the funded coalitions. Ideas such as Plan4Health work to improve access to healthy foods and promote physical activity such as walking and biking as transportation options. Unfortunately, rural communities are not likely to benefit from these types of partnerships.

Health disparities connected to the way the environment is planned and built will endure in rural Appalachia unless we pay attention to the specific conditions within this region. It is ridiculous for many rural communities to talk about installing bike lanes when, like Forest County, Pennsylvania, they are still trying to manage their sewage. Furthermore, Appalachian residents in rural areas are not concerned about separating residential from commercial or industrial land uses; the economy has done this for them. The public health issues in Appalachia may appear similar to the rest of the country, but additional environmental health concerns related to the built environment are more pressing here. Added to these concerns is the need for land-use planning decisions to be the main economic development tools in many local places. Overall, the built environment plays a profound role in the inequities that have contributed to health disparities in Appalachia.

3

A Place for Water

I believe water quality is the number one priority. It will not get
any cleaner or more abundant. We must find innovative ways to
ensure water quality for future generations. My county is very
poverty-stricken. Many of the poverty-stricken homes have antiquated, sometimes open bored wells. Some even have old hand-
dug wells. Approximately 50 percent of all bacterial water samples
result in a positive sample for total coliforms and *E. coli*. We have
very little public water in a five-hundred-square-mile county.

—Appalachian environmental health professional

Every well in rural Kentucky is contaminated with sewage.

—Appalachian environmental health professional

WYOMING COUNTY, WEST VIRGINIA, IS TUCKED INTO THE
southern corner of the state in the Appalachian Mountains. It is promoted
as the "hidden gem of southern West Virginia."[1] The Wyoming County
Economic Development Authority describes it as "rich in both history and
natural beauty. Rushing brooks; mighty mountains; and wild, wooded areas
make up its rugged topography, with small communities and three diminu-
tive municipalities—Mullens, Oceana, and Pineville—dotting the landscape."[2]

More than forty years ago, I would visit my cousins in the hills of Pineville, and now I am revisiting the area with a fresh perspective. My childhood memories of Pineville have blurred with time, but I was oblivious then to coal's impact in the area, even though my uncle worked for Joy Manufacturing, a company that makes mining equipment.

One small community in Wyoming County embodies an environmental health reality prevalent throughout Appalachia. Bud, West Virginia, is one of numerous places relying on an ailing drinking-water system built by coal mine owners in a rush to locate their workforce close to their mines. These systems were meant to be temporary, useful until the companies were done taking all the coal and closed the mine, so they were built with little regard for the environment or health. But after mines near Bud began to close, people stayed in this company town and the community is now defined as a census-designated place. It is not incorporated as a village or town, but it is recognized as a "settled concentration of population."[3]

The population of Bud in 2015 was 440 people, down from the 487 recorded in the 2010 census. The 2010 census indicates that almost 40 percent of Bud's residents live in poverty. The median household income (MHI) in Bud was $18,571, less than half the MHI for the state of West Virginia and about one-third the MHI for the United States. Most of the homes in Bud were built in the 1970s. The median housing value of $9,999 ranks lowest in the state. There is one K–8 public school in Bud that feeds students to two high schools in the county. A little more than two hundred kids attend the school, and for more than six months in late 2013 and early 2014 they could not drink the school's water. While the media, the public, and politicians focused on water problems in Charleston, West Virginia, resulting from the January 2014 spill of chemicals into the Elk River, the rural community of Bud in coal country had been struggling for months without access to clean, safe water.

A privately owned, family-run system supplied water to the school and surrounding community of Bud. The Alpoca Water Works system was so neglected by the owners that, in a January 2013 letter, the state Office of Environmental Health Services identified it as a "serious health concern."[4] The warning letter also explains that the water system "most likely was established decades ago by a coal company to serve a local coal camp community." This system was the sole source of drinking water for the residents of Bud, including the school. In other places it is somewhat unusual for public drinking water to be supplied by a private company, but the coalfields of Appalachia are different than other places.

To protect public health, state and local environmental health officials negotiated with the owner to take control of the system. While negotiations were underway, the residents of Bud were left with no alternatives for their water.

Environmental health officials issued a boil order for Bud's water in September 2013. For the next several months, there were days when people in the community, including the school, could not use their water at all, even if it was boiled. The water system was dangerously contaminated and did not comply with regulations designed to protect public health. In January 2014, the EPA published a formal enforcement notice for the system because there had been no monitoring to ensure that the water was safe to drink. The boil order was finally lifted in April 2014 after the local public service district bought the water system, hired an operator, completed deferred maintenance, and tested the water. After more than half a year, the residents of Bud could finally drink their water. In a statement to the press, State Senator Mike Green underscored the relative status of water resources in rural communities when he said, "I know the Charleston water crisis made national headlines, but the scope and duration of this event affected the residents of Wyoming County as much or more than the Elk River situation."[5]

The story of drinking water in Bud is not unusual in Appalachia.[6] It reflects a long history of environmental neglect and, in some cases, outright abuse, much of it tied to coal mining. Since 1912, when the first mine opened within its limits, King Coal ruled Wyoming County. Coal was the key source of jobs in the county for decades; it brought both prosperity and people to Appalachia. For the people who live in many small places, when it comes to environmental health, coal's positive impacts are waning while its negatives are waxing. Since 1990, almost half of the coal mining operations and more than half of the mining jobs have disappeared from Wyoming County. Even so, about a thousand people still work in active underground mines in the county and are taking millions of tons of coal from them.[7] The active mines are obscured by remnants of closed underground mines and rusted coal conveyor belts that dot the landscape.

Despite still mining millions of tons of coal every year, workers in Wyoming County have suffered the same fate as those throughout West Virginia. Their jobs were built on the state's natural resources, first timber, then coal. At its high point in the late 1940s and early 1950s, more than 120,000 people worked in coal operations in West Virginia. Since then, there has been a steady decline in coal employment. In 2013, a little more than 52,000 people were employed in the industry, almost 31,000 of whom were identified as independent contractors, a job classification that limits health and other benefits to miners.[8] As employment in mining decreased, the overall state unemployment rate increased. The unemployment rate in West Virginia hit double digits in the early 1990s, peaking at 11.6 percent in January and February 1992.[9] This was the same time that coal employment sunk to its lowest levels.

Employment in West Virginia began a rebound in the late 1990s, but the recovery was undone in 2008 as the country headed into a recession. The state's unemployment rate doubled between 2008 and 2010. Unemployment in Wyoming County was more severe than the rest of the state during this same period, jumping from 4.7 percent in 2008 to 10.3 percent in 2010.[10] Unemployment and poverty tend to follow the same path. This path has led the people in Wyoming County to one of the highest poverty rates in a state with one of the highest poverty rates in the country.[11]

It is still harder to find a job in Wyoming County than in other parts of West Virginia and the county's unemployment rate remains high.[12] There are few alternatives to coal, and county residents and elected officials seem to have been unable to imagine a future without it. Since coal was the main source of jobs for decades in most of West Virginia, many local places are still struggling to recover from the loss of these jobs. Coal's legacy includes more than just economics, however: environmental and health concerns are left in its wake as well. In local places, like Bud in Wyoming County, where coal was the sole source of prosperity, its legacy now seriously degrades both human and environmental health

Unemployment and poverty are two determinants of health and can partially explain why Wyoming County, West Virginia, ranks among the lowest in the state for health outcomes and health factors.[13] Data reported by the Robert Wood Johnson Foundation's County Health Rankings program reveal that 27 percent of adults in the county say they are in fair or poor health. Overall, the county ranks 53rd out the 55 counties in West Virginia based on indicators that negatively affect health. These factors include health behaviors such as smoking, obesity, and physical inactivity. One in four adults smoke, more than 40 percent are obese, and more than one-third of adults surveyed said that they do not participate in any leisure-time physical activity. Interestingly, in the county described as the gem of the state at least in part because of recreational activities, more than one-quarter of the residents say they do not have access to exercise opportunities such as parks.

Health behaviors, access to clinical care, and social and economic factors are vitally important to overall health status, but environmental health factors embedded in place are equally important. Safe drinking water is a crucial place-based determinant directly affecting public health. In numerous locations throughout Appalachia, when the coal industry declined, it left behind more than just persistent economic issues; it also contaminated water and created current drinking-water problems such as those found in Bud.

APPALACHIAN WATER

In the water resources of Appalachia you can find some of the most important aquatic species in the country. They are also the reason that Appalachia is considered a center of biodiversity and a national environmental treasure.[14] Clean drinking water from underground aquifers and mountain springs has been abundant enough for people to settle in areas far removed from any public water supply. In some places all it takes to have access to drinking water is a bucket and a nearby spring. If you do not live near a mountain spring, you might dig your own well to get to your drinking water. While the quantity of water may be plentiful in Appalachia, the quality of water is much less certain. Numerous factors affect water quality in the region, but the combination of inadequate infrastructure and deep-rooted environmental contamination creates challenges that seem insurmountable in some places, especially those holding on to hope that coal will make a comeback.

Even as coal mining has declined in Appalachia, past practices continue to plague current water quality. Abandoned or inactive underground mines are the most important sources of acid mine drainage and the Mine Safety and Health Administration estimates that there are more than three hundred thousand abandoned mines in Appalachia.[15] When water accumulating in these mines is released, accidentally or on purpose, it usually contains high levels of an iron compound. As this water meets air, a chemical reaction occurs to create sulfuric acid and dissolved iron. The water looks orange or yellow because of the iron content. The acid lowers the pH of local streams and creeks, wiping out entire ecosystems and rendering the water too dangerous to drink. Because of the long history of coal and the numbers of abandoned mines, many of which's locations are unknown, acid mine drainage is a distinctive Appalachian problem.

Adding to the historical environmental assaults from mining are the contemporary assaults from natural gas drilling, train derailments, storage tanks, untreated sewage, and aging or nonexistent water infrastructure. The numerous offenses to water quality in Appalachia are already a major concern because of their environmental consequences and the potential impacts on ecosystems. However, human exposure to degraded water supplies is arguably the most important public health issue in Appalachia because of the wide range of human-made and natural pollutants and systemic weaknesses in handling these pollutants.

Many of the activist environmental organizations working in the Appalachian region focus on chemical contamination of water supplies, specifically concentrating on water impacts related to coal and natural gas drilling. Multiple incidents compel their activism. This is especially the case when serious high-profile incidents, such as the Elk River chemical spill, affect drinking water for thousands of people. When an event of this magnitude occurs, it captures the attention of politicians and others who declare "never again." In fact, there are numerous places in Appalachia that are less likely to be affected by a major chemical spill than by bacteria contaminating water due to failing septic systems. What is perhaps an even more sobering reality than these acute contamination incidents is that some small communities in the region have chronic problems with access to safe drinking water.

WATER INFRASTRUCTURE

Even with an abundance of water resources, places in the Appalachian region lack adequate infrastructure to provide safe drinking water and treat wastewater. In some instances, Appalachian people are contaminating their drinking-water supplies with their own waste. Every time they flush the toilet, they send contaminants into their source of drinking water. I saw firsthand how this happens during my first week on the job with the Ohio Environmental Protection Agency (Ohio EPA) in the early 1990s on a site visit to Appalachian Ohio. Three small, rural communities were under enforcement orders to address their sewage treatment problems. At that time, all three communities were relying on private systems maintained by individuals. In some households within these communities there was no system at all. When people flushed their toilets, wastewater went directly to ditches in front of their homes. Eventually the communities partnered to install sewers and a wastewater treatment system with the technical and financial assistance of Ohio EPA. Nevertheless, the images of raw sewage in people's front yards have stuck with me for more than twenty years. This circumstance introduced me to the challenges that rural Appalachia faces when it comes to improving environmental health conditions, especially in relation to water quality.

Even in places with access to good water, there are not always the means to manage water after it is used for drinking, bathing, cooking, or washing clothes. There are entire small communities in the region in which wastewater is straight piped directly into a ditch or stream. Environmental health professionals in Appalachia are frustrated by their lack of resources to address this untreated wastewater. They routinely express concerns about failing private septic systems and their inability to call attention to how microbiological pathogens make people sick. Their frustration is compounded by public outrage and resource priorities that focus on the water quality impacts of chemical spills. This focus leaves many rural places to fend for themselves to solve the problems associated with untreated sewage. Because of low population densities, rural areas are less likely to have access to sewers, so people who live in these areas manage their own sewage. Distances between communities combine with physical characteristics of rural places to make public wastewater collection and treatment prohibitively expensive.

According to the 2017 American Housing Survey, about 18 percent of the total occupied housing units in the United States use onsite, private systems for managing their wastewater.[16] This is good news because it means more than 80 percent of households are served by public sewers and treatment facilities. Properly functioning public facilities minimize environmental health impacts from wastewater. These are places where sewers collect and transmit dirty water to treatment facilities before it is released into the environment. These facilities are mostly publicly owned treatment works or POTWs. POTWs hold permits from regulatory agencies that set limits on contaminants in treated water. They are expensive to build and require constant maintenance and monitoring. When these systems fail, the environmental health impacts can be catastrophic.

In general, the public water infrastructure in the United States is crumbling with age and inadequate maintenance. Declining tax revenues for upgrades and maintenance, uncertainties in federal grant and loan programs, and shifting public health priorities make it challenging to maintain, expand, or build new treatment plants and sewers. Among the most visible impacts of aging wastewater infrastructure are the hundreds of combined sewer overflows (CSOs) threatening public health in hundreds of places in the eastern United States.

These threats exist particularly in Pennsylvania, Ohio, and West Virginia and are often found in smaller communities of less than ten thousand people.

Combined sewers consist of one pipe that carries both storm water and wastewater from residences, commercial sites, institutions, or any other structure in a community. When it rains hard, as it often does in Appalachia, the combined sewers cannot handle all the water and they overflow. Sometimes the pressure during an overflow is so great that manhole covers can jettison skyward. CSOs bypass treatment plants or exceed their capacity, and raw sewage ends up floating in rivers, ponding on streets, or filling up basements. When people encounter this contaminated water during a flood event, they confront a serious health risk from pathogens and other substances.

Water infrastructure is challenging for several reasons, regardless of whether it is public or private. Private infrastructure is essentially self-regulated, with minimal, if any, oversight from public health authorities. Local health officials are responsible for monitoring private systems and their ability to do this is tied to available resources. In resource-poor areas, septic systems and drinking-water wells often operate for decades without inspections and problems are not identified unless there is a complaint or a real estate transaction. In most states, private wastewater systems are required to connect to a public system if sewers become available. On the other hand, property owners are generally not required to tap in to public drinking water. The health impacts of contaminated drinking water on one property will be minor compared to the potential public health impacts of a failed septic system.

The Appalachian Regional Commission has been working to improve both drinking and wastewater infrastructure for more than fifty years. One of the ARC's main objectives for improving regional economic conditions has been to upgrade and increase infrastructure. Water infrastructure is an important component of economic development and the ARC has provided funding for drinking-water and wastewater projects. However, unlike the highway system, there is no dedicated pot of money for water infrastructure in Appalachia. This means Appalachian states compete with others for a diminishing share of available federal funds for water improvements.

At first these funds were part of a construction grants program through the Clean Water Act. In 1990, Congress ceased appropriating funds for grants and created the State Revolving Loan Fund. This loan fund is administered by states, and local governments typically acquire funds through a competitive process. Additional federal agencies provide funding for water system improvements, including the Departments of Agriculture, Housing and Urban Development, and Health and Human Services, but the State Revolving Loan Fund programs are the largest source of funds specifically targeted toward improving systems that treat drinking water and manage sewage.

The shift from grants to loans has destroyed the ability of public health professionals to prioritize specific projects in Appalachia. In addition, because the loan program requires repayment from communities, it severely reduces the capacity of water improvements in the region. These loans, as well as operating and maintenance expenses, are paid through monthly service fees by residents. Rural communities are at a serious disadvantage when it comes to planning, installing, and maintaining water infrastructure in terms of both technical and financial resources.[17] The loan program raises questions of equity because it effectively discriminates against some places despite their overwhelming need for the improvements the loans can provide.

In the case of wastewater, property owners will likely pay a connection fee of thousands of dollars for access to the public sewer. Even though there are some grants and low-interest loans available to individuals, this can be an insurmountable financial burden to people who are living below the poverty line. Furthermore, when a new public system is installed, the expenses are shared by community members, so the smaller the population, the greater the debt burden per individual. Changes in federal funding have led to a situation in which, in the words of one study, "significantly fewer households in Appalachia have access to centralized drinking-water and wastewater services than households in the rest of the country do. On a per capita basis, documented infrastructure needs for Appalachia are on par with the rest of the country. However, the financial capacity of households and communities to meet those needs lags significantly behind the national average. As a result, households in Appalachia with access to centralized systems pay a much higher percentage of their income for water and wastewater services than households in the United States as a whole do, on average."[18]

The ARC has paid attention to water infrastructure, but its focus has always been on the economic benefits of enhanced infrastructure, rather than the public health costs and benefits. Safe drinking water and improvements in wastewater services for individual households may not seem like an economic development issue, but improving public health has the potential to lead to positive economic impacts as well. When people are healthy, they do not miss work, they need less access to the health care system, and their overall quality of life improves.

Regardless of the economic benefits, safe water is one of the most effective ways to protect and promote public health. Public health should be a major goal for any organization dedicated to regional development, and addressing public and private water infrastructure is a means of accomplishing this goal.

DRINKING WATER

The source of drinking water is dependent on place, and Appalachia's residents obtain their drinking water through both public and private systems. A public water system is defined by the Safe Drinking Water Act as one that serves at least twenty-five people (or fifteen connections) for at least sixty days per year. Even though public water systems are classified based on the number of people they serve, it is difficult to get a precise measure of the actual population with access to these systems. This is because a system at a large facility, such as a university or hospital, might serve thousands of people who are not residents of the state in which it is housed. Thus, sometimes the total population served by public drinking-water systems exceeds the state's total population. For example, according to the Safe Drinking Water Information System (SDWIS) managed by the EPA, Alabama's public water systems served more than 5.5 million people in 2013.[19] The total population of Alabama that year was estimated at 4.9 million. Using geography to estimate people supplied with water from public systems paints an inaccurate picture of drinking-water access in most states. The SDWIS makes it appear that 93 percent of Appalachia's population is being served by public water systems. This is likely a gross overestimation because of how this data is compiled.

Regardless of the size and classification, all public water systems are regulated by the government. This means that they must comply with federal and state laws and regulations designed to protect public health from exposure to a range of contaminants in the water. Unlike public drinking-water systems, those served by individual private drinking-water systems, such as residential wells, are using water that is not regulated. In these instances, it is up to consumers to test their own wells. Unregulated private systems can expose people to contaminants that are never documented or corrected by environmental health professionals. The absence of reliable estimates regarding the numbers of people who use private water systems is troubling. These systems often pose the greatest health risks to low-income people who live in rural or remote places, such as Bud, West Virginia, but they are not on the radar of public health officials the way large public systems are.

In addition to the type of treatment system, the source of drinking water influences its safety. About one-third of the public water systems in the United States are served by groundwater and the remainder use surface water as their source. Surface water includes rivers, ponds, lakes, and human-constructed reservoirs. Both surface and groundwater can become contaminated through a wide range of legal and illegal activities. In most cases, however, it is more challenging to protect groundwater from pollution than surface water.

Groundwater is contained in underground rock formations known as aquifers, and the United States Geological Survey monitors the quality and use of the nation's main, or primary, aquifers. There are several primary aquifers under the Appalachian states. A primary, or principal, aquifer is a "regionally extensive" underground source of potable water.[20] Most of the groundwater in Appalachia is contained in the Appalachian Plateau, a system of aquifers predominantly consisting of sandstone near the surface with shale and coal below. One of the largest sandstone aquifers in Appalachia is identified as the Pennsylvanian, which encompasses sections of Pennsylvania, Ohio, Tennessee, New York, Kentucky, Alabama, and West Virginia. The Pennsylvanian is a sandstone aquifer with a shallow depth to the groundwater, so it relies on rain and snow to recharge. The shallowness of the aquifer also makes the groundwater susceptible to contaminants from the surface and safeguarding the land is critical to maintaining safe drinking water.

In sparsely populated areas of rural Appalachia, those who use private systems for drinking water are more likely to use groundwater than surface water. Once groundwater is polluted, cleaning it up is expensive and involves technology that might take years to be successful. A variety of sources can contaminate groundwater, including septic systems, industrial accidents, and underground drilling and storage activities. Getting attention when small communities like Bud are suffering from the effects of unsafe drinking water is not easy. On the other hand, chemical contamination of water supplies serving less rural areas becomes national news. Prioritizing urban over rural areas can be an obstacle to public health improvement in Appalachia. Then again, whenever a major environmental tragedy befalls the region it brings to light the unique environmental health challenges found in Appalachian places.

Elk River Becomes a National Place

The ruptured tank that caused a drinking-water disaster in 2014 is located a few feet up a steep slope from the Elk River near Charleston, West Virginia. The site had been used for petroleum storage since the late 1930s and was locally owned until the 1970s. At that time, it was sold to Pennzoil-Quaker State for storing waste motor oil. In 2001, Pennzoil-Quaker State sold the facility and the new owner removed the petroleum products and transitioned to storing chemicals, largely used by the mining industry. Since 1990, state regulatory authorities conducted multiple inspections of the facility under the authority of the Clean Air Act. Likewise, inspectors regularly performed hazardous waste compliance checks . Conversely, for several years leading up to the spill, there was no indication of any inspections for compliance with the Clean Water Act.[21] A 2009 internal inspection of the facility indicated that the tanks contained glycol solutions and calcium chloride. Inspection records do not note the chemical that caused the panic in Charleston, MCHM (4-Methylcyclohexanemethanol), in any of the tanks.

Freedom Industries bought the site in December 2013. Freedom Industries incorporated in 1992, but the company that existed in January 2014 was a combination of four different companies. The spill was discovered on January 9, so it became known as the Freedom Industries spill. Records gathered by the West Virginia attorney general's office indicate that, because of the smell and public complaints, it is likely the chemical had been leaking from the site for some time.[22] This means chemicals from the main tank could have been oozing into the groundwater below it well before local people began smelling it.

The extent of contamination to groundwater has not yet been determined and the long-term public health consequences are still unknown and unknowable. Alarmingly, there has never been a human health assessment of MCHM. The dangers from the lack of risk information about the chemical are further compounded by the fact that there is no specified regulatory enforcement level for the maximum amount of MCHM in drinking water. The EPA sets maximum contaminant levels (MCLs) for hundreds of substances in drinking water, including microbes, radionuclides, disinfection by-products, and a range of chemicals. There was no MCL for the licorice-smelling chemical MCHM in the Elk River spill, at least initially, and MCHM was not the only chemical in the contaminated water.

With no human exposure data and no information from the EPA about MCHM, the Centers for Disease Control and Prevention quickly established a level based on information in fact sheets provided by the chemical's manufacturer. The CDC then requested that the National Toxicology Program (NTP) conduct studies to address uncertainties associated with human exposure to

MCHM. The NTP is housed in the National Institute of Environmental Health Sciences in the National Institutes of Health, and the program is responsible for conducting research on substances with potential human health effects. The NTP completed a series of short-term tests using several of the chemicals found in the Elk River spill and determined that the exposure levels hastily set by the CDC were protective of human health. In June 2015, the NTP released the results of its research and the director of the CDC's National Center for Environmental Health was paraphrased as stating in a radio interview that the "NTP study results confirm the determination in the early days of the spill [by both the CDC and the Agency for Toxic Substances and Disease Registry] that the levels of MCHM in drinking water were not likely to be associated with adverse health effects."[23]

The federal environmental health tests were important steps in managing the spill, but they were probably little comfort to the hundreds of people who went to hospital emergency rooms with headaches, nausea, and rashes. An accidental spill of chemicals affecting drinking-water sources is not an unusual event. If ever there was a case to spotlight the antiquated regulatory system that is supposed to ensure the safety of chemicals used in coal mining, Elk River is it. The fact that there was and still is so little information about the public health consequences of exposure to the substances in this spill forecasts an ominous future for Appalachian communities that are harboring remnants of mining.

Buoyed by the public outcry over the MCHM spill, in late 2015 the US House of Representatives revised the 1976 Toxic Substances Control Act (TSCA), also known as the Frank R. Lautenberg Chemical Safety for the 21st Century Act.[24] The TSCA requires companies to test and register chemicals to ensure that they do not pose public or environmental health risks. MCHM was being used at the time the TSCA was ratified in 1976, so it is one of almost eighty-five thousand chemicals grandfathered from requiring compliance with the law. As with many unfunded mandates, regulatory oversight of chemicals under the TSCA has been lax. In addition, we have developed tens of thousands of new chemicals since 1976 and the EPA is unable to ensure the safety of most of them before they are introduced into the marketplace. The Lautenberg bill became law in June 2016 with President Barack Obama's signature.

If Congress follows through and provides adequate resources to implement the law, the Elk River spill could serve as a catalyst for meaningful reform and this accident could mean that Appalachia is the place that made the rest of the country just a little bit safer. The 2016 election weakened the potential impact of these revisions to the TSCA. It seems as if protecting the environment and public health is no longer the mission of the federal government and implementing the Lautenberg Act is likely to be one of the casualties of this change in tone and approach. The head of the office at the EPA responsible for regulating chemicals has clearly indicated that the agency's priorities will focus on keeping chemicals in the marketplace, regardless of what the scientific community says about their health risks.[25]

FROM DRINKING TO WASTE

Everyone understands the importance of safe drinking water to keeping people healthy, but managing water containing human and other wastes is crucial to improving and maintaining public health as well. Wastewater treatment removes physical (solids), chemical, and biological contaminants from water before it is dumped back into the environment. Inadequate wastewater treatment contaminates local and regional drinking-water sources, damages ecosystems, and causes negative health effects. Wastewater management was the first place-based public health approach and laid the foundation for the environmental and public health professions. So, long before science connected the dots of germs to disease, people realized the importance of the environment and place in preventing illness.

Wastewater management was at first mainly a question of collecting contaminated water and moving it away from people to minimize exposure. Communities dumped raw sewage into ditches and waterways, and people did not think twice about it because they could not smell it or see it. Eventually, as urban populations grew and human settlements clustered into historically unimaginable densities, just moving untreated wastewater away from people was not enough. Engineers and scientists developed methods to use natural filters to remove contaminants from the water.

Soil was the most available filter. The earliest wastewater treatments systems were designed to allow dirty water to percolate through the soils. Experiments using soils as filters combined with pipes to transmit the filtered water took place in the late nineteenth century. By 1892, twenty-seven American cities provided some form of wastewater treatment.[26] Treatment technology has evolved considerably since the 1890s, but the basic process is still the same, relying extensively on filtration. Eventually wastewater operators began to disinfect the water as a final step in the treatment train. These processes ensure that harmful biological organisms are minimized in the water returned to local streams, rivers, and lakes. Many contemporary wastewater treatment plants use chemicals such as chlorine and bromine for disinfection, while others use ultra-violet radiation.

As with drinking water, both public and private systems manage waste-water. Sewers are the foundation of functioning public systems and they are expensive to install and maintain. Generally, sewers use gravity to transmit waste-water to a treatment plant, but this depends on the terrain and the geology of the place being served. The reliance on gravity also means that public treatment plants are best located at a low point in the community to minimize the need for pump stations. Once the sewage reaches the treatment plant, the facility must have the capacity and technology to ensure clean water. The expense of installing and maintaining public systems often hamstrings rural communities from solving the environmental health problems associated with untreated sewage.

Wastewater Treatment Needs in Appalachia

The EPA conducts a Clean Watersheds Needs Survey (CWNS) every four years as part of the requirements of the Clean Water Act. The CWNS compiles information about public wastewater systems and assesses capital needs for these systems. This survey does not focus on operation and maintenance needs after these systems are constructed.[27] States submit data for the assessment, relying on their regulatory records and information provided by local operators. The EPA reviews and compiles the data to estimate how much money is needed to install or upgrade public wastewater systems. Not all states participate in the survey and many rural areas and small communities are likely not well represented because they lack capacity to provide data for the report. Nevertheless, in 2012 the estimated financial needs for twelve of the thirteen Appalachian states amounted to almost $25 billion, accounting for more than 35 percent of the needs for the entire country.[28] This was a slight increase in the estimated needs from the 2008 assessment. According to the CWNS, more than four thousand wastewater treatment facilities in twelve Appalachian states need improvements. Almost one-third of the systems in Appalachian states serve communities with less than a thousand people.

The CWNS does not address operation and maintenance of these facilities, which can be expensive and unaffordable to small communities. In most instances, even small facilities require a certified operator to be available twenty-four hours a day, and finding qualified individuals in remote locations is not easy. Beyond all these logistical issues, it is also important to remember that it is not sustainable to build new treatment plants without funds for operating and maintaining them. When public treatment systems fail, there can be devastating environmental and health consequences. Minimizing the potential for these failures requires resources for keeping these systems in good working order.

Addressing public wastewater treatment is important in Appalachia, especially as a potential economic development strategy. What cannot be overlooked, however, is the impact of failing septic systems on the health and well-being of the region.[29] Rural areas in Appalachia have some of the highest concentrations of bacteria in their drinking water. At least some of this contamination is connected to inadequate treatment of wastewater in these areas. As with private drinking-water wells, it is almost impossible to accurately estimate the number of private septic systems. The best we can do is estimate the percent of the population served by public systems and then assume that the remainder are using some sort of private method to manage their waste. Septic systems are "undocumented" and "unidentified" needs in the region.[30]

When people cannot access public treatment works, septic or other types of private systems are the alternatives. Septic systems are simple in design and easy to maintain, but homeowners must be educated about their operation and maintenance. The most basic system consists of a large concrete tank and a series of plastic pipes. Water that includes solids is flushed from the housing unit into the tank, where solids settle to the bottom. Water exits the tank through pipes to the leach field, which distributes it into the soil. This water seeps into the ground to be treated by natural microbes in the soil of the leach field. Soil type is the most important environmental factor ensuring that septic systems will work effectively. Soils must be able to filter out pathogens while allowing the water to percolate without pooling or ponding.

Depending on the soil type and drainage characteristics, a well-maintained septic system is a good solution for many rural areas. However, since many rural homes have both private drinking-water wells and septic systems, it is critical for the wastewater system to be separated from drinking-water wells. Many states mandate minimum distances between the two. In addition, some states have minimum lot sizes for private systems to ensure that there is enough space for the leach field. None of the minimum regulatory requirements make any difference to the older systems that are dotted throughout the rural areas of Appalachia. Regulations also do not affect the multitude of straight-pipe systems that are still associated with the coal camps of the early twentieth century.

Back in Wyoming County, West Virginia, there are portions of five distinct coalfields and several coal camps within the county boundaries.[31] According to a 2009 report, about 85 percent of the land in Wyoming County is owned by companies from outside of the county. Much of this land contains remnants of coal camps that housed miners and their families almost a hundred years ago.[32] Most of the coal camps did not install sewage collection systems. Rather, pipes sent dirty water directly into rivers and creeks. Some of this straight-pipe discharge of wastewater is still happening in Wyoming County, and untreated household sewage is still polluting local water bodies.

One of the greatest challenges with private wastewater treatment is educating individuals about the importance of maintaining their current systems, in addition to fixing problems that may compromise their water quality. Both education and maintenance take resources, and resources are scarce in Wyoming County. As with many of the local rural health departments in Appalachia, there is one full-time environmental health specialist in Wyoming County, and this person is responsible for protecting the public's health from diseases spread by food, air, waste, vectors, and water. This imbalance between responsibility and resources exemplifies water management in Appalachia and has created and will maintain environmental health inequities and health disparities in rural Appalachia for years to come.

4

A Place for Food

Everybody had a garden but we didn't have one 'cause I lived with my grandmother and she was a domestic worker, in the house cleaning, washing. So we didn't have a garden but our neighbors had a garden so they gave us food. . . . There was a grocery store when I was young. This [pointing] was a grocery store and then the big attorneys, they closed it up. There was a store up there where the new business is now, and a store down there where the restaurant is. And at one time over there where the garage is was a store, too. So, we had a lot of little stores. And they started disappearing after the war when people would get tires and gas and go to the city and shop in the Kroger Supermarket.

—Eighty-five-year resident of Athens County, Ohio

ABOUT ONE IN THREE PEOPLE IN ATHENS COUNTY, OHIO, LIVE in poverty. It is the poorest county in the state.[1] It is also one of thirty-two counties in Ohio designated as part of the Appalachian region of the state. Even in the face of poverty, Athens County has a lot going for it, especially when it comes to food. On Saturdays, you can find a large crowd at one of the best farmers' markets in Ohio. Restaurants in the city of Athens, the county seat, boast of using local suppliers for many of their menu items. The Convention and Visitors Bureau highlights the county as being "home to one of the nation's first 'super-local' food economies" with the program known as the "30 mile meal."[2]

A range of organizations and initiatives enhance the local food economy and many of these assist local entrepreneurs in starting their own food-related businesses. Even the major public university in Athens includes local foods as part of the supply for the dining halls.

Despite all these initiatives and activities, the Food Environment Index compiled by the Robert Wood Johnson Foundation (RWJF) ranks Athens County dead last among the eighty-eight counties in Ohio for access to food.[3] The RWJF combines measures of food availability and food security to generate the index, including two specific measures: (1) how close low-income people live to a grocery store and (2) how many people did not have reliable access to food in the previous twelve months. People in rural areas who lack physical access to food live more than ten miles from a grocery store. Reliable access to food is an indicator of financial barriers to obtaining food. Athens County has the most limited access to healthy foods and the highest level of food insecurity in the state.

The USDA Economic Research Service (ERS) gathers much of the data used in the Food Environment Index. However, the ERS's Food Environment Atlas paints a more comprehensive picture than the index does of place-based food challenges.[4] The atlas includes a wide range of statistics, such as the availability of fast food restaurants and retail grocery stores, food assistance programs, and average prices of some common foods. According to the atlas, more than 23 percent of Athens County residents lived more than ten miles from a grocery store in 2015. As in many rural areas, most of the people in Athens County who lack physical access to a grocery are also low-income. People in rural Athens County travel long distances to purchase what little food they can afford.

A major public university in Athens County accommodates more than twenty thousand students, faculty, and staff from August through May. The university both complicates and enhances the county food environment. On the one hand, students may be counted in some of the food environment indicators, which could be distorting data. On the other hand, the university contributes to the success of local food initiatives by providing a base of customers who are educated and opinionated about food choices. Regardless of how the university affects the local food environment, it is an island in a sea of poverty in southeastern Ohio. Its location sets up interesting and contradictory scenarios related to food access, especially with regard to local foods. Emphasizing local foods will not solve problems of physical or economic access for many year-round Athens County residents, but it does appeal to faculty, some students, and visitors. Local foods, especially those steeped in Appalachian culture, are clearly used to promote tourism and as tools for economic development.

The Appalachian food culture has been a function of poverty for decades. Looking back, you can find poverty's influence in the agrarian society that was once common in Appalachia. People living in remote areas needed to be self-sufficient, so they farmed, hunted, and fished to feed their families. Some of the foods most associated with Appalachia, including ramps, pawpaws, pork, and venison and other game animals, are parts of this historical culture. Contemporary food culture is also tied to poverty. However, now poverty has led Appalachians to abandon the farm and head to the Walmart. People rely on foods that are low cost in terms of dollars spent, but high cost in terms of the public health consequences. As the traditions of subsistence farming and hunting fade away, new, equally cost effective, but less healthy means of sustenance have arisen.

Appalachian staples such as ramps and pawpaws are still part of the region's food culture and you can find local festivals dedicated to these and other foods. The annual pawpaw festival in Athens County draws thousands of people every autumn to taste a wide range of concoctions made with this fruit. Pawpaws and other foods are also now part of the local food movement. As such, their importance and cultural resonance in the Appalachian diet has seemingly shifted from feeding the poor to accommodating the middle class. The Appalachian foods that saw many people through hard times are now for sale at inaccessible farmers' markets rather than inexpensive Walmarts. There is a food paradox in Appalachia because, while it is the home of an abundant variety of native fruits and vegetables, it is also a place where many people struggle to afford fresh, healthy food.[5]

INSECURE FOOD

Food security is "access by all people at all times to enough food for an active, healthy life."[6] Researchers and governmental agencies categorize food security as high, marginal, low, and very low. Households categorized as high and marginal are considered "food secure" because there is little or no disruption in their normal diet. Food-secure households generally have consistent access to food, even though there may be some anxiety about having enough for their next meal. On the other hand, households categorized as low or very low are identified as "food insecure" in terms of both food quality and quantity. Those households in the very low category experience hunger at times and often cannot buy enough food or create balanced meals. People in the very low category will skip or cut the size of their meals.[7] Very low food security used to be labeled "food security with hunger," but this changed in 2006. Even though the government removed "hunger" from the definition, it is not removed from the circumstances of these households.

Recall that Athens County, Ohio, has the highest rate of food insecurity in the state. Let's explore one factor of the local food environment: access to grocery stores. The county had twelve grocery stores and twenty-eight convenience stores in 2014.[8] In 2019, there are nine Dollar General stores within twenty miles of the city of Athens. This means it is easier for Athens County residents to access convenience stores than grocery stores, just based on geography. Getting to a convenience store might not require using gas for a long drive over winding rural roads. As convenience stores increase in number in rural areas, local grocery stores decline. Local grocery stores are further doomed when large discount retailers set up shop. Rural places attract major food retailers because they have adequate space for stores with thousands of square feet and hundreds of parking spaces. These supercenters keep their prices low by purchasing high volumes from suppliers so they both create and fill a void in some places.

Food insecurity is prevalent in rural places and rurality might even be an indicator of its presence.[9] Measures of food insecurity in Ohio pinpoint counties with major urban places, such as Columbus, Cleveland, Toledo, and Cincinnati.[10] However, food insecurity concentrates in the more rural counties in the Appalachian region of the state. This pattern of food insecurity is found throughout the states in the Appalachian region. Urban places typically have high rates, but rural places tend to have the highest rates. Furthermore, food insecurity is increasing in rural areas even as it decreases in much of the country.[11] You can look at the empirical data to confirm this, or you can drive by the local food pantry and see for yourself. People might struggle every day to find enough food to be healthy, even when there are programs that could assist them.

One such program is the Supplemental Nutrition Assistance Program (SNAP), formerly referred to as Food Stamps. SNAP is the largest governmental program that addresses food security, providing monetary benefits to more than 36 million low-income people in the country. Even though SNAP is a federal program, states have flexibility in administering it. This includes determining who is eligible for benefits. Eligibility is based on multiple demographic factors, including income, employment, and disability status. Eligibility is also based on an individual's or household's current assets and expenses. People may be eligible to receive benefits, but that does not mean they apply for them, and very few states have 100 percent participation of eligible households.[12] The fact that not all eligible people participate in SNAP contributes to underlying concerns about food security because it suggests that this assistance program is not helping some of the people it is designed to serve.

Those who do participate in SNAP can use their benefits to purchase healthy foods. However, geographic access to groceries seems to be more difficult for rural SNAP participants than urban participants.[13] In addition, something unexpected is being observed among SNAP participants. In general, their overall health is not improving. Specifically, SNAP beneficiaries are a little more likely to be obese than those who are eligible but do not participate.[14] As public health researchers explore the relationship between obesity and food access, they are raising questions about why those who are most food insecure tend to be overweight or obese. To put this another way, people who worry the most about their next meal, people who are often hungry, and those who may skip meals to make the food last longer, are more likely to be obese than people who do not suffer from these problems.

Almost 30 percent of the urban population in the United States is obese or has a body mass index (BMI) of 30.0 or higher, while about 43 percent of the rural population is obese.[15] This is a significant difference in obesity rates between rural and urban places. It rounds to about one out of every three people in the United States being obese regardless of where they live. The problem of obesity is glaring in Appalachia, as it consistently has some of the highest rates in the country. In 2018, West Virginia, the only state entirely within Appalachia and one of the most rural states in the nation, had the highest obesity rate in the country.

Many factors influence obesity. Food security is one determinant, and the relationship between food security and obesity is particularly prominent with children. Child food insecurity rates are substantially higher in rural places than urban places.[16] Children who experience either low or very low food security are more likely to be obese.[17] Nationwide rates of childhood obesity have increased at an alarming rate since the early 1970s. According to the National Health and Nutrition Examination Survey, childhood obesity has more than tripled since

1974.[18] Five Appalachian states have the highest obesity rates among high school students. Young people in West Virginia, Kentucky, Tennessee, South Carolina, and Georgia are among the most obese in the nation.[19] Furthermore, obesity rates have been increasing steadily for more than a decade, to the point where almost 20 percent of high school students are considered obese. This epidemic of obesity is connected to important health conditions among youth, including high levels of diabetes and cardiovascular disease.[20]

This is what we know about food security in Appalachia: (1) several states in Appalachia are among the least food secure in the country; (2) within these states, rural areas tend to be less food secure than urban areas; and (3) Appalachian states post some of the highest overall and childhood obesity rates in the country. All these disparities exist within a region with a seeming abundance of healthy food options that include community-supported agriculture, farmers' markets, and a renewed emphasis on local foods. The health outcomes related to food security appear to be based less on the food and more on the interrelatedness of place and poverty, two factors that arise repeatedly as the most important targets of any strategies to improve public health in Appalachia. In the meantime, some think that improving access to local foods will help solve the problem of food security.

LOCAL FOOD PLACES

Farmers' markets, community-supported agriculture (CSAs), and community gardens revolve around promoting local foods. Beyond these, a local-foods movement that includes retailers from roadside stands to Walmart is also a piece of the Appalachian food's scene. The movement is buoyed by increasing consumer demand for a variety of reasons, including concerns about improving local economies, protecting the environment, and enhancing nutrition. Whether local food initiatives will contribute to solving the problems of food insecurity and safety in Appalachia is uncertain. However, it is worth talking about the growth both in farmers' markets across the region and in some food-related diseases such as diabetes.

There are positive aspects emerging from the local-foods movement and the upsurge in interest in farmers' markets, especially when it comes to efforts to increase overall access to fruits and vegetables. The numbers of farmers' markets in the United States is expanding exponentially. Unfortunately for the people of Appalachia, especially those who live in rural areas, these markets may not be increasing their access to nutritious and local foods. The number of markets listed with the USDA has dramatically increased since 1994, when 1,755 markets were on the list. In 2019, 8,771 markets were on USDA's list, with more being added almost weekly.[21] Most of these emerging markets are in urban and suburban areas where they can accommodate people who want locally grown products and enthusiastically support them. In addition, urban farmers' markets are often found near large grocery stores in order to attract as many customers as possible.[22] This strategy increases foot traffic at these urban markets because people may shop for staples at the grocery and local products at the market.

Urban markets, especially those near grocery stores, provide service to higher-income people and thus attract more farmers and vendors than is the case in rural areas with a sparsely distributed population. Rural markets face obstacles in finding accessible locations and in encouraging local farmers to participate as vendors. Multiple competing influences result in fewer farmers' markets serving low-income people in rural areas than those that serve more affluent urban or suburban places. Indeed, there may be an inverse relationship between food assistance programs, such as SNAP and electronic benefits transfer (EBT), and access to farmers' markets.[23] Reiterating the point about challenges with physical access to food, those who could reap the greatest benefit from access to a farmers' market often live the furthest away from them.

The USDA directory categorizes farmers' markets by market location type, such as private business parking lots, local-government building grounds, educational institutions, or closed-off public streets. These locations offer a general sense of the additional inequities between urban and rural locations of farmers' markets. The USDA listing identifies markets that are "on a farm: a barn, a greenhouse, a tent, a stand, etc." Although this is an extremely rough estimate with a lot of assumptions, the USDA list identifies less than 1 percent of markets as being in the category of "on a farm."[24] However, in looking at a map of where these "on the farm" markets are located, none are in West Virginia, Tennessee, or Kentucky. In Appalachian states with this type of market, such as Ohio, Maryland, Virginia, North Carolina, and Georgia, few are in the Appalachian-delineated counties. Physical location is one of the main reasons why rural people cannot access farmers' markets. An additional access barrier is the limited hours the markets are open, with some only open for a few hours every week.[25]

For farmers' markets to make a difference in food security in Appalachia, it will take significant resources to conveniently locate markets that are open during accommodating hours, stocked with fresh produce, and able to accept food assistance for purchases. Allocating resources to do this to address food security and its associated health issues is risky because the relationship between access to farmers' markets and lower rates of obesity is still unclear.[26] While farmers' markets may conjure images of tables and stands full of fresh and healthy produce, a significant percentage of products tend to be non-produce items. In one study in an urban setting, almost 40 percent of the products for sale at twenty-six farmers' markets were processed items such as baked goods and jams.[27] Even setting this research aside, farmers' markets cannot compete with most grocery or convenient stores in terms of hours of service and variety of foods, further inhibiting their ability to serve as alternatives to these existing retailers.

Farmers' markets are incredible resources for local economies. They provide access to homegrown products and they offer opportunities for local growers to make some money for their hard work. A sense of community also inevitably evolves as consumers and farmers interact over food. The positive aspects of farmers' markets are many, but addressing social justice issues related to food security is not one of them. As a matter of fact, farmers' markets may have enhanced food injustice due to simple supply-and-demand economics. That is, they may have made it possible for rural farmers to take their produce out of local places to areas with a higher number of potential customers. This could mean that people in rural places lack access to foods that are grown in their communities.

The societal impacts of farmers' markets are one facet of a system that includes two food aspects that affect health in Appalachia, namely security and safety. While food security is related to chronic health conditions such as obesity, food safety is associated with more acute health outcomes, including those that make it difficult to work, study, or play. Diarrhea, vomiting, and nausea are seemingly minor conditions in comparison to hunger and malnutrition, but collectively they have a major societal cost. Places lacking capacity to promote food safety are subject to negative health outcomes arising from one of the most preventable environmentally related exposures. Even if farmers' markets are not a panacea for food security, they will remain an environmental health issue for food safety professionals because they fall in the realm of facilities requiring adequate resources for regular monitoring and inspection.

SAFE FOOD PLACES

As with most environmental health programs, every state manages farmers' markets differently, even though most states require a permit or license for vendors. With the tremendous increase in the number of farmers' markets, local health departments are facing even greater demands in ensuring that food is safe for consumers. The regulations governing farmers' markets generally correspond to the type of foods being sold. For example, eggs usually must be kept under refrigeration during transport and sale. Meats and cheeses are also subject to temperature controls. Many states do not allow the sale of home-canned goods or baked goods that are made in home kitchens. Some stalls at markets are required to have hand-washing stations, especially when meat or poultry are being offered for sale. Then, there is a litany of regulations around the marketing approach of offering samples to consumers, including specifications as to the type, amount, and timing of samples. Adding to the regulatory scheme is a transient vendor base, changing the nature of the markets from week to week. All these regulations, and often many more, are implemented by local environmental health professionals who must inspect the markets and evaluate their compliance. The complexity of ensuring food safety at farmers' markets only adds more tasks to a workforce that is often already stretched too thin.

What makes food unsafe in Appalachia? Unlike factors influencing food security and many other environmental health problems, there are no foodborne pathogens unique to the region. Appalachian people are as likely as others to be exposed to *Salmonella*, *E. coli*, noroviruses, and other familiar bacteria and viruses. Where inequities arise in terms of food safety in Appalachia is in the ability of people in the region to prevent and respond to foodborne illness. A central function of environmental health practice is controlling the contamination of the food supply, and food safety inspections are a significant activity in most local health departments. Even though there is broad federal food safety legislation involving numerous state and federal agencies, the local sanitarian protects the public from foodborne illness. In many rural places, this means that a single sanitarian is responsible for ensuring food safety along with managing every other environmental health matter that could affect public health for hundreds of square miles.

The elements contributing to the incidence of foodborne illness are well known. They include improper cooking and holding temperatures, poor personal and employee hygiene, and food from unsafe sources. Continual oversight and education are necessary to minimize the impact of these factors. Oversight comes in the form of local resources to enforce food safety regulations and education involves in-depth training of those who process, serve, and sell foods. The circumstances surrounding unsafe food are common across the country, but the economic conditions in Appalachia may hinder the ability to control even well-known factors that make food unsafe. In rural Appalachia, sparse public health resources greatly factor into the risk of suffering from foodborne illness.

Finding resources for environmental health is challenging in the best of times, but when resources are tight, it is even more so. Many federal public health agencies, including the CDC, are subject to budget cuts on a regular basis.[28] In the face of austerity, federal, state, and local governments must identify and address public health priorities that may be shifting daily. The most prominent problems are often tied to public perception rather than scientific evidence. Examples such as bioterrorism or Ebola virus in the United States create a great deal of public attention and require public health officials to dedicate significant resources to addressing concerns. In other cases, new priorities emerge and change from fiscal year to fiscal year. Daily prevention activities collapse in local places as resources are diverted from such tasks as inspecting restaurants to dealing with controlling the spread of substance abuse. Public health agencies will almost always have limited funds to accomplish unlimited tasks, so sometimes decisions are made based on immediate societal costs and benefits, rather than longer-term population health effects.

In terms of food-related public health issues in Appalachia, addressing diabetes and obesity are priorities. I find it difficult to argue that these are not major public health concerns based on the evidence. Yet we cannot overlook the fact that focusing on diabetes and obesity draws attention and resources away from food safety and toward food security and nutrition. This means that food-processing and retail inspections are often underfunded and understaffed in resource-poor places. Food insecurity is a vital determinant of public health, but environmental health professionals are generally more involved with food safety than security, specifically in preventing people from getting sick by eating unsafe or contaminated foods. Food-related outbreaks are more likely to result when facilities are not adequately monitored by environmental health professionals. It is somewhat paradoxical, then, that attempting to address food security and boost nutrition with farmers' markets has increased the food-safety burden on local health departments.

Even though food safety is a fundamental component of environmental health, foodborne illnesses still affect millions of Americans every year. The CDC estimates that about 48 million people suffer food poisoning annually, about 128,000 people become so ill they have to be hospitalized, and perhaps as many as 3,000 people die as a result of something they ate.[29] Most of the documented illnesses are related to bacteria and viruses—or microbes—that can find their way into foods anywhere along the route from the farm to the table. Microbes are especially concerning because of their ability to adapt to environmental changes. The CDC monitors outbreaks of and trends regarding pathogens in foods and has documented the rise of microbes resistant to tried-and-true treatments. Some strains of *Salmonella*, for example, are now resistant to several antibiotics. Other microbes are beginning to show up in places not traditionally part of their environmental range. Microbes, especially bacteria, are highly sensitive to temperature, so it is likely we will see more pathogens in unusual places as average temperatures rise with climate change.

The national reporting system documented more than 16,000 foodborne outbreaks in the thirteen Appalachian states between 1998 and 2017, accounting for more than one-third of all outbreaks in the country during this time period.[30] That averages out to about 1,200 every year in the region or almost three per day. An outbreak is defined as foodborne illness involving two or more people linked to a common pathogen, location, or food. Additional data from the CDC for the Appalachian states indicate that more than 93,000 people became ill during that time period and more than 3,100 of those may have died from foodborne illness. These foodborne illness data are alarming, but we need to interpret them with some caution. These data are reported for entire states, including major urban centers outside of the region like New York City and Baltimore, Maryland. On the other hand, foodborne illness is notoriously underreported, so there might be more outbreaks than are currently documented. The last time you had diarrhea, did you call the local health department to report your illness?

A group of viruses known as norovirus and several species of *Salmonella* bacteria are the pathogens most often implicated in outbreaks in Appalachian states. These two microbes account for more than 50 percent of the documented outbreaks and contribute significantly to the burden of disease linked to consuming unsafe food. A variety of foods can harbor these bugs, including salads, produce, gravies, seafood, cheese sauce, turkey, and even cake. As might be expected, the largest documented outbreaks, those that cause the most illness and death, are tied to retail or institutional food service rather than private homes. This fact doesn't mean eating away from home is more likely to make you sick. People do not contact local public health officials when they make themselves or their family sick by mishandling food.

Noroviruses are a public health threat because they are hardy, ubiquitous, and can spread in multiple ways, including through food. It is common for noroviruses to contaminate food when those preparing or serving it do not wash their hands properly. Outbreaks of norovirus in Appalachian states have been connected to a wide variety of foods and places. From a salad bar at a school in Georgia to a banquet facility in Mississippi, and in fast food restaurants throughout the region, noroviruses are everywhere. Each year, hundreds of thousands of people get sick from ingesting these viruses in their food. Food-related norovirus is just the tip of the iceberg when it comes to the impact of this pathogen on public health. This group of viruses is linked to many other outbreaks, including those on cruise ships and other places of leisure and recreation. The Appalachian Trail is a unique source of norovirus.[31] Hikers may not have adequate access to clean water for waste management or hand washing. When hikers leave the trail and head into small towns and villages, they can bring the virus with them and start the spread of illness in the local places that accommodate them.

Aside from noroviruses, *Salmonella* bacteria are especially problematic. They are among the most common causes of foodborne illness in the United States, affecting millions of people every year. There are more than 2,700 different strains of *Salmonella* bacteria and new ones continue to emerge. So, while outbreaks are often reported as just *Salmonella*, environmental health investigators attempt to identify the specific strains of the pathogen involved. *Salmonella* is often implicated in major, multistate outbreaks, such as several notable incidents involving alfalfa sprouts, peanut butter, and chicken. Until recently, these multistate outbreaks were often linked to large farms or food processing facilities. However, two outbreaks may offer some foreshadowing of the impact of local foods on illness.

In 2015, CDC reported 252 people in forty-three states became infected with one of five strains of *Salmonella* that were linked to live poultry in backyard flocks.[32] Of these cases, 141, or about 55 percent, were identified in the Appalachian states, with Ohio leading the pack. The sick people who were interviewed told the CDC they purchased the live poultry so they could raise their own eggs, meat, and pets. In each case, the illness emerged after having contact with live poultry. This situation opens a new realm of possibilities not even on the radar several years ago. Managing food safety issues will surely continue to evolve raising more concerns about the lack of resources for monitoring and responding to foodborne illness.

Perhaps it was one of these backyard flocks that contributed to a *Salmonella* outbreak in Watauga County in Appalachian North Carolina in the summer of 2014. The restaurant that was the source of the outbreak was not a chain, and the menu featured a statement about their commitment to local food sources. The local health department estimated that about forty people got sick, and it was likely that the eggs used to make crab cakes caused the illnesses. In a letter to the editor of the local paper, the owner of the restaurant noted that they use both local and grocery-store eggs and that it was not possible to determine which eggs caused the problem. Even so, she made the commitment to continue to support local farmers in their restaurant. Like the backyard flock outbreak, this restaurant outbreak linked to locally sourced foods further exemplifies new challenges for environmental health professionals in preventing, monitoring, and tracking food outbreaks.

Backyard flocks and other home-grown products create an interesting scenario in Appalachia. These products, along with farmers' markets, might lead to additional disparities between wealth and poverty and urban and rural places in the region. The restaurant in North Carolina is not likely to be a place where people living in poverty would go to get a meal. Farmers' markets catering to a wealthier clientele are out of reach to people who do not have access, governmental assistance, or other financial resources. Could the local-foods movement be making richer people in urban Appalachian places as sick as food insecurity does in rural areas? This question is not easily answered, but it needs to be raised because this is where local health departments without power and influence specifically affect those with power and influence. Since food safety is a major component of environmental health practice, it is also a significant portion of the budget for many public health agencies. Consequently, as the resources for food safety are contracting, circumstances leading to foodborne outbreaks are expanding.

SAFE AND SECURE FOOD

Making Appalachia a place where all people have reliable access to safe food is not going to be easy. Several activities show some promise in addressing food security and safety in underserved areas, including Appalachia. Family food assistance programs, initiatives targeting food nutrition labeling, enhancements to local food sources, and changes to school lunches are partial solutions to some of the food-related health problems. These initiatives will need to emphasize safety as well as nutrition in order to mitigate the burden of foodborne illness, because healthy foods are not only high in nutrients, they are low in pathogens.

Schools are among the most important places to monitor and enhance good practices that will ensure safe and secure food. Schools are also the places where some of the most vulnerable people are exposed to multiple health threats daily. Food insecurity was one of the cornerstones to the establishment of early school lunch programs after research documented the impact of hunger on learning.[33] In 1946, Congress passed the National School Lunch Act to provide states assistance in serving meals to their residents based on their financial need. The strategy of supporting states based on income data is still the foundation for federal appropriations for school lunches. However, in the 1960s legislation modified the funding formula and the amount of money sent to states was cut. The National School Lunch Act has been amended by Congress multiple times since 1946 but retains its focus on meeting minimum nutritional requirements and supporting states in funding programs for local school districts with the most need.

The legislative intent of providing lunches to needy children has remained at the center of federal assistance to local places. Participation rates in school lunch programs are particularly useful in assessing poverty because they provide data by school district, something that the United States Census does not do. The federal government uses household income data to determine whether a child is eligible to receive free or reduced meals. These eligibility standards, which are related to federal poverty levels, are supposed to be updated every year.[34] In order to participate in the program, individual families must apply to their school, detailing household income including both earnings and public assistance. Families receiving SNAP or other food benefits are automatically eligible for reduced-price or free lunches.

Over time, the percentage of school-age children in the United States who are eligible to receive free or reduced-price meals has steadily increased. During the 2013–14 school year, 52 percent of public school students were income-eligible to receive a free or reduced-price school lunch, a more than 10 percent increase from the 2000–2001 school year.[35] Since eligibility requirements change annually and are based on federal poverty rates, the increase in eligibility suggests that more school-age children live in poverty now than they did fifteen years ago. In looking at data for individual states, nine of the thirteen states in Appalachia have more eligible children than the total US rate. Mississippi has the highest rate in the country. More than 72 percent of the school-age children in Mississippi are eligible to receive a free or reduced-price meal in the national school lunch program.

Even though there is evidence that children who participate in the school lunch program eat a healthier diet than those who do not, the overall quality of the diet of school-age children in the United States is lacking.[36] This came into focus with First Lady Michelle Obama's attempts to improve children's health by modifying the national school lunch program. In 2010, she led the charge to change nutrition standards for school lunches for the first time in fifteen years.[37] The new standards included mandates that school lunches provide more fruits, vegetables, and low-fat milk and reduce the amount of sodium and trans-fat. The intent of the changes was to address the increasing rates of childhood obesity in the United States

At first, there was widespread support for this approach. Public comments related to the proposed rule were overwhelmingly in favor.[38] Then, in 2014, several organizations joined the US House of Representatives in calling for more flexibility in the rules because of their possible costs. The School Nutrition Association (SNA) argued for "relief from some of the onerous regulations slated to take effect this summer, which will lead to fewer students receiving healthy school meals, more food being thrown away and many school programs in financial straits."[39] In fact, SNA's position specifically in opposition to increasing availability of fruits and vegetables continued to perplex healthy food advocates in 2015.[40] The costs of improving the school lunch program are seen as too high today, even though this preventive approach could minimize billions of dollars in healthcare costs in the future. The work of Michelle Obama was essentially wiped out in 2018, when the USDA issued a final rule to give schools more flexibility in determining their lunch menus.

Working on providing nutritious lunches in schools addresses food security but leaves food safety on the sidelines. Serving unsafe fruits, vegetables, and proteins can lead to illness that also interferes with learning. Schools account for a small percentage of foodborne outbreaks every year, but they should concern parents and educators alike. The CDC compiles data related to outbreaks at the state level, so it is not possible to specially identify outbreaks in Appalachian counties, and using data for a state like New York would likely make the problem look more intense than it is. However, using West Virginia for illustration purposes, there were thirty-nine outbreaks located in schools from 1998 through 2017.[41] More than 2,800 people, presumably many children and young adults, became ill during these outbreaks. These statistics raise additional questions about the impact of foodborne illness and the capacity of environmental health to prevent their spread.

FOOD PROGRAM CAPACITY

Capacity is an issue for both food security and safety in Appalachia. Even though there is potential to address food security in Appalachia by using many governmental programs already in place, there are challenges to overcome. These challenges include reaching those most vulnerable to food insecurity to encourage their participation in these programs. Once enrolled, it may be necessary to monitor participants to ensure that quantity of food does not supersede the quality of food. Considering the relatively low levels of enrollment in food assistance programs, additional strategies to improve food security could include more attention to using local foods in ways to benefit low-income people in rural areas.

Public support for efforts to make school lunches healthier can also chip away at food insecurity by adding to the reliability of fresh, wholesome foods. However, public support is not enough when special interest groups get involved in determining what is on school lunch trays. Even if we are able to provide more nutritious foods in school cafeterias, it does not mean that children will eat better. The access to healthier foods must be combined with incentives and efforts to educate children and families about the benefits of eating healthier. The capacity to provide this education is questionable in school districts struggling to meet testing benchmarks. Yet for many children, school is the one place where they can get a nutritious meal that can build the foundation for their future.

Athens County, Ohio, is a compelling case study of the convoluted and often contradictory nature of food-related health disparities. It also offers an example of the many facets of food safety and security in a rural area of Appalachia. The county has the highest rates of poverty in the state that is ranked among the lowest in the country for per capita spending for public health activities, including for environmental health.[42] The county has an active, lively local-foods movement, but poor people do not have reliable access to healthy, nutritious foods. Grocery stores are closing, while the convenience and supercenter food stores are thriving. More than one-third of the adults in the county are obese and about one in ten has diabetes. There is one health department in the county that covers both the city of Athens and the county as a whole. There are only a few full-time sanitarians at this health department responsible for all the restaurants, farmers' markets, schools, food trucks, and every other food processing or service facility in the county. Their service area includes eighteen cities and villages covering more than five hundred square miles and more than sixty-four thousand people. The best way to ensure that food is safe in this specific county and Appalachia in general is to make it an environmental health priority.

5

A Place for Pollution

We are people who have worked at the plant when it opened and
are still alive. They . . . it's not killing people. Yes, there are some
people who have gotten cancer from their own stupidity. I know
that from asking enough questions when stuff got declassified.
You got neighbors and family that work out there and will tell
you that some people were given and were using safety appara-
tus and would remove it. Just to smoke a cigarette, while they are
still using a cutting torch on a pipe that's letting off green fumes.

—Local Appalachian county economic development director

People first and foremost are concerned about jobs and to a
large extent that's the reason you find a lot of people in that area
who are happy to have the plant there, and are willing to bring in
a nuclear reactor because it means jobs, or at least they think it
means jobs.

—Resident of Appalachia, Ohio

PIKE COUNTY IS IN THE HEART OF APPALACHIAN OHIO, A
landscape of both scenic rolling hills and farms sprawling across the flatlands.
It is a rural county about one hour south of Columbus and forty minutes from
the Ohio-Kentucky border. The county seat is Waverly, with a population of

92

about 4,300 people. The Pike County Convention and Visitors Bureau promotes Ohio's "most perfect tree," a two-hundred-year-old maple, and the county's connection to the Ohio and Erie Canal as reasons to visit the area. Pike County also houses a 3,700-acre nuclear facility currently being managed by the US Department of Energy (DOE). The Portsmouth Gaseous Diffusion Plant, or PORTS, is one of three places in the United States that enriched uranium for the military to use in nuclear weapons during the Cold War. The site, which is currently undergoing an immense cleanup operation, is referred to as the "A-Plant" (A for "atomic") by Pike County residents and those who live nearby. The A-Plant presents a thought-provoking case study of the environmental health legacy of facility siting in Appalachia, and it raises questions about how and why rural places are chosen for large-scale, potentially dangerous facilities.

In the early 1940s, the Atomic Energy Commission (AEC) began a process of identifying places to enrich uranium needed by the Department of Defense. The AEC was attracted to rural areas that offered large, inexpensive tracts of land, proximity to existing road and energy infrastructure, and extensive access to water resources. In addition, it was reasoned that an accidental release of radioactive material would have less impact in areas with low population densities. The AEC selected two places in Appalachia, one in Oak Ridge, Tennessee, and one in Pike County, Ohio. A third site, in Paducah, Kentucky, is not part of the officially designated boundaries of the Appalachian region, even though much of Kentucky is.

Pike County's geographical location was just one factor in the decision to build the plant there: another was access to a competent labor pool. While the federal government was selecting locations for these facilities, a workforce analysis identified an ample supply of workers within commuting distance to the Pike County site.[1] The rich supply of labor was due to a decline in industry in the area, which led to a high rate of unemployed skilled workers. Construction of the A-Plant began in 1952 and, at its 1954 peak, 20,749 people were employed at the site.[2] Considering that the total population of Pike County in 1950 was only 14,607 people, these construction jobs were immensely significant to the economy, creating a boom for adjacent counties. Suddenly, jobs were abundant not only in Pike County but throughout southeastern Appalachia Ohio.

In 1956, uranium enrichment was fully underway at PORTS. Times were good. Entire families worked at the plant. People wanted to live near the A-Plant, even knowing some of the risks, because they were content with well-paying, patriotic jobs. These high-paying jobs with great benefits and retirement plans were rare in a place with locally persistent poverty and high unemployment rates. PORTS powered the economic engine in this rural area, making Pike County a desirable place to live for decades. Meanwhile, the purpose of enriching uranium was transitioning from nuclear defense to nuclear energy in the 1960s to support a period of growth in nuclear power in the United States. Many were hopeful that nuclear power would become a viable alternative to coal. The federal facilities that produced weapons-grade nuclear materials assumed a prominent role in producing nuclear fuel for electricity generation. The first nuclear power plant went online in 1958 in Shippingport, Beaver County, Pennsylvania, an Appalachian place discussed further below.

At first, people viewed generating electricity with nuclear fuel as an economic benefit. Shifting priorities from defense to energy meant that uranium enrichment would continue and jobs at facilities such as the A-Plant were safe. Pike County maintained a strong economy, based almost completely on the plant and the businesses supporting it. Positive attitudes about nuclear power began to change in the late 1970s, however. In 1979, the movie *The China Syndrome* was released as a fictional, but accurate, portrayal of a disaster at a nuclear power plant. The nuclear power industry was not helped when there was a partial meltdown of a nuclear reactor at Three Mile Island in (Appalachian) Pennsylvania, twelve days after the movie hit theaters. The fictional and real dramas catalyzed activists and contributed to the birth of a social movement. In 1982, an estimated one million people participated in an antinuclear protest in New York City. Politicians could not ignore the fact that attitudes about nuclear power were no longer positive.

It is not likely that any of the workers at PORTS drove to New York City to participate in the 1982 march. What is likely is that the march and the meltdown at Three Mile Island created local economic impacts in Pike County, including a significant loss of jobs at the A-Plant. It took less than thirty years for uranium enrichment to descend from patriotic darling to environmental enemy. Nuclear power plants were no longer welcome in many communities, despite their promise for job creation. The average age of commercial nuclear power plants in the United States is now approaching the forty-year mark.[3] Even though there are a few new plants under construction or planned, it is almost impossible to garner public support for nuclear power. The market for enriched uranium declines every year and natural gas extraction is accelerating this decline.

One consequence of siting massive federal facilities in small rural communities is that they quickly dominate the local economy by providing numerous high-paying jobs to people who have few alternatives. The economic dominance creates a combination of dependence and fear as community and individual livelihoods revolve around these hazardous plants.[4] People are grateful for jobs with benefits, but they might also be concerned about negative public health, environmental, and occupational impacts. As PORTS was being built, laws related to facility siting and operations that would require attention to occupational and environmental health were still more than twenty years in the future.

Congress created the EPA in 1970, as the country was reacting to multiple events that underscored the environmental health effects of uncontrolled pollution. Four years after the creation of the EPA, Congress replaced the AEC with the Nuclear Regulatory Commission (NRC). The NRC now regulates construction and operation of nuclear facilities. While the government was creating agencies and implementing policies to improve worker and environmental health, the A-plant kept on enriching uranium, discharging pollution, and endangering workers.

Congress did not enact environmental laws addressing many aspects of nuclear sites until the early 1980s. These laws included the Comprehensive Environmental Response, Compensation, and Liability Act (CERCLA), which contains the Superfund program to provide money for cleaning up hazardous waste sites. Federal facilities, such as PORTS, were exempt from the law until Superfund was reauthorized by Congress in 1986.[5] After that, places owned by the US government were required to adhere to the environmental laws required by all other industries. The environmental health circumstances at PORTS surfaced when the status of federal facility compliance with environmental laws and regulations changed.

In 1989, the State of Ohio filed a civil action with the DOE requesting that the judge affirm an agreement to clean up PORTS. The agreement, or consent decree, focused on ensuring the "safe and environmentally sound handling of hazardous waste, mixed waste, PCBs, solid waste, and water pollution."[6] Despite decades of enriching uranium on the site, environmental monitoring data showed that the main environmental health issues were not related to radioactive substances. Rather, PORTS is contaminated with organic chemicals used and stored at the facility. Many of these chemicals have been found in the groundwater. Those in charge of cleanup at PORTS identify the main priority as ensuring the contaminated groundwater does not migrate off the site. If it does, it might affect the drinking-water wells of residents in the area. Since the cleanup did not begin until shortly after the 1989 agreement, area residents and plant workers could have been exposed to contaminants for more than thirty years.

Large-scale uranium enrichment at the facility ceased in 2001 and by 2005 cleanup was the main activity at the A-plant. The decline in uranium enrichment led to a decline in local jobs. There was a 38 percent decrease in private, nonfarm employment in Pike County between 2000 and 2009. During this same time period, the state of Ohio experienced only a 10.8 percent decline in employment. During the cleanup, a consulting firm employs about two thousand people at the site under a contract with DOE. Much of this employment does not promise to be long-term, since it is funded largely through temporary government sources, including the American Reinvestment and Recovery Act and grants and contracts from the DOE. In addition, with each congressional budget negotiation, people worry that funding will be cut or completely terminated.

Once a hub of activity related to national defense and then a promising site for nuclear power development, Pike County is now experiencing business closings, family exodus, and economic despair. The unemployment rate is creeping up and the county is consistently among the highest in the state for job loss. Employment numbers in Pike County and other Appalachian places do not tell the story of how many people move to find work, nor do they explain what happens to the people who are left behind. Leaving the place that has been your home for generations because there is no work is heart-wrenching to some families who have deep roots in the area. Those who remain in Pike County are subject to poverty, unemployment, lack of access to health care, an emerging epidemic of drug use, and environmental health inequities. In 2019, Pike County made national news when a middle school closed because radiation was detected inside the building.[7]

Pike County is consistently ranked among the lowest of Ohio counties for health factors overall, and social and economic factors specifically.[8] Pike County is not unique in the social and behavioral determinants contributing to poor health. The one thing that makes Pike County different than every other county in Ohio is the A-plant. Even with concerns about environmental health and a great deal of anecdotal evidence about cancer perceived to be connected to the plant, people who live in the area still support PORTS because it continues to provide a solitary hope for jobs.

Pike County and its experience with the A-plant exemplifies the struggle in Appalachia to improve the economy while protecting environmental and public health, a balancing act that has become fundamental in the region. Why is it that Appalachian communities have been the destinations for so many major polluting industries and environmental activities that degrade the region and affect public health? As in many other places in Appalachia, the presence of the A-plant in Pike County does not explicitly prove that pollution causes poor health. Establishing this causal relationship will continue to thwart environmental health researchers for the foreseeable future. It took decades to prove that cigarettes cause cancer, and that was a direct, visible, and (mostly) voluntary exposure. Showing associations between environmental contamination and health is a more daunting task. The fact that there are multiple scenarios like the one in Pike County, throughout the region, clearly suggests a need to further examine the connection between the location of polluting facilities and the health status of people nearby. One certainty is that, from a strictly geographic perspective, some of the industries and activities that emit the highest levels of pollution have found a place in Appalachia.

LOCATING PLACES FOR POLLUTION

Imagine I own a waste management company and I am looking for a place to build a new landfill. Because my company is profit-motivated, I must find the most economical location. From my business's perspective, the best sites are going to be in areas with large tracts of cheap land. It is a plus if these areas are already serviced by infrastructure such as water, roads, and electricity. In addition, there should be an ample supply of skilled workers who are desperate for job security. With these things in mind, there is a giant welcome mat in rural Appalachia.

Before I start construction, I must acquire permits and comply with regulations for siting and operating a landfill. These regulations mandate where the landfill can be located and how the landfill is designed and operated.[9] Some of the regulations limit places for me to build the landfill. I cannot build near an airport because birds flock to landfills, causing airplane accidents. I could look at sites that are in floodplains as long my landfill would not interfere with natural flooding or cause waste to be released during a flood. On the other hand, my landfill is not allowed in a wetland, unless a state environmental agency makes an exception. Geologically sensitive areas, including fault zones and seismic impact areas, are also restricted from consideration.

Even though landfill restrictions do not specifically rule out locating a facility over a primary source of drinking water, many of the explicit construction requirements are designed to protect groundwater. Both upstream and down-stream groundwater monitoring wells are required for detecting if pollution is leaking through the bottom of the landfill into the groundwater. If a leak is detected, the mandatory liner in place to stop liquids from seeping into the ground has probably been breached. The liner is usually a combination of clay and a synthetic material for catching liquid at the bottom of each landfill cell. The liquid, or leachate, is then pumped out of the bottom and usually treated to make it less hazardous. The environmental regulations for landfills are one example of how the government can constrain site selection. These regulations apply to new landfills built after 1984. All the places that handled waste prior to that time were essentially unregulated and many have become hazardous waste sites because of this.

Federal laws and state regulations for facility siting, whether for landfills, power plants, or other potentially hazardous sites, should contribute to finding locations most protective of the environment and health rather than those that are most expedient. Even with regulations, the ultimate factor in locating many facilities is often local public support or opposition, more so than finding the place most suitable for practical or technical reasons. This means that promises of vigorous economic impacts can be prime motivators for selecting sites. Decisions to build potentially hazardous facilities are often based on politics, not policy. Decision makers seek to gain public approval and get reelected, rather than prioritize public and environmental health. Throughout Appalachia, high unemployment rates have contributed to the facility-siting decisions of developers, elected officials, and people who live in economically distressed communities.

The historical emphasis on solving economic, rather than health or environmental, disparities in Appalachia has resulted in many places being inundated with potentially harmful industries and activities. People hear their elected officials promise new jobs, or to save existing ones, and they rally around facilities even if it means relaxing local environmental regulations. Communities then become havens for pollution from which they reap few economic benefits but many environmental health costs. There is a "pollution-haven hypothesis" (PHH) which suggests that American corporations target specific places in other countries for polluting facilities because of lax or nonexistent environmental regulations.[10]

The existence of pollution havens implies that decision makers intentionally select places for hazardous activities for reasons not related to operational and technical suitability. In these cases, facility-siting decisions are the result of overt environmental injustice. Industries find their home where poor people and minorities live because these communities are marginalized, eager for jobs, or both. Pollution havens can exist within countries, not just between them.[11] If a place has high levels of pollution without correspondingly high levels of economic rewards, it might be a pollution haven. This includes places with factories, power plants, refineries, and other facilities employing relatively few people, considering their environmental impact.

To pursue this line of thinking, delineating the presence of a pollution haven within a country involves identifying "pollution-per-economic reward" indicators.[12] One example of this type of indicator is calculating the amount of pollution released for every job tied to the polluting facility. This is an imperfect statistic because of limitations with the data, but it nevertheless offers estimates of the relation between the environmental and the economic impact of polluting facilities. It also allows for comparing places based on relationships between amounts of pollution and numbers of jobs. Picture a large facility that reports millions of pounds of pollution released to the air and water but does not employ a significant number of people. In this case, the ratio of pollution per job would be high, suggesting that the environmental health costs are greater than the economic benefits. When this ratio is combined with indicators of wages, enforcement activities, and other factors, possible pollution havens emerge in rural counties, including Pike County, Ohio.[13]

Environmental injustice exists in places where there is lax enforcement of regulations. Often, we can identify these places by looking at socioeconomic characteristics such as race and income.[14] Using enforcement activities to indicate pollution havens in the United States is tricky, because all states are required to comply with the same federal environmental laws and regulations. Differences emerge because state and local governments have some latitude in writing and enforcing regulations, provided theirs are not weaker than federal ones. The policy of requiring state regulations to be at least as stringent as federal law should promote economic parity among places. State governments cannot promise weak environmental compliance as a bargaining chip to encourage new industry within their borders. State and local governments turn to other strategies such as tax breaks and zoning laws to compete for facilities in the name of economic development.

Generally, local governments have freedom when it comes to land-use decisions. This autonomy was made clear in 1926 when the US Supreme Court validated the use of zoning as a legitimate use of police power.[15] In this case, the village of Euclid, Ohio, was trying to stop a developer from building multifamily homes and commercial enterprises on property he owned. The developer argued that a new zoning ordinance forbidding his plans violated his constitutional property rights. The Supreme Court decided that the village's ordinance was constitutionally valid because it served a legitimate public purpose, including a "relation to the public health, safety, morals, or general welfare."[16] The Euclid case set a precedent for local zoning ordinances now commonplace around the country. While these ordinances can focus on separating land uses to abate nuisances, they also encourage or discourage land uses, including those that create environmental hazards. Local zoning regulations contribute to pollution havens because they are essentially place-based regulations that can lead one community to accept an environmental health hazard, while another bans the same. It is the "general welfare" that is open to local interpretation and provides the foundation for allowing some land uses because of potential economic benefits.

Local officials are motivated by economic development opportunities when making land-use decisions. This is especially important when local jobs are scarce, since the impacts of unemployment ripple through the community, affecting schools, infrastructure, and social services. An unemployed skilled workforce leads to a positive and supportive political climate for facilities that would not be welcome in many communities. Corporations seek these types of places to exploit local economic conditions as a means for garnering public support. When jobs are scarce, places are vulnerable to exploitation and may even compete for new industry as a solution to high unemployment rates. Because of their economic despair, people who live in some of the most impoverished places offer their support for activities that promise to provide an immediate job. Their short-term needs are so great they are unable to weigh environmental health costs to the community against the economic benefits for their families, and they may actually fight to get hazardous facilities built.

A bidding war occurs when places vie for new facilities for the sake of immediate economic benefits. Local merchants envision the influx of workers as a boon to their business and small governments anticipate the impact of additional tax revenue. These larger-community economic impacts cannot be ignored by politicians who must respond to pressing issues affecting their constituency. Landfills, power plants, chemical manufacturers, and hydraulic fracturing have cropped up across Appalachia in places where local officials go out of their way to encourage and welcome any kind of economic development, whatever the risks. After the competition between communities to build these facilities is over and the elected officials have moved on to other matters, the winners may see a temporary burst in jobs. What community residents may not foresee is a future when their victory will seem like a defeat; when, for example, their grandchildren suffer from high rates of cancer, asthma, and developmental delays.

In many ways, locating a place to build a polluting facility is not complicated. It involves finding enough land and adequate infrastructure, but land and infrastructure are available in rich places as much as they are in poor ones. This suggests that factors other than capacity and feasibility are more important. In some places, residents join elected officials to fight for facilities to solve local economic problems. The question of whether their economic problems are actually solved is rarely answered because, to answer this question, we must look at how exposed people benefit or suffer from their proximity to pollution. Using the "pollution-per-economic reward" approach is one way to investigate inequities in exposures that are not tied to jobs. When we take this approach, we can find many places in Appalachia where the promise of jobs has been the primary factor in locating large-scale projects that have large-scale environmental health impacts.

JOBS AND POLLUTION

Going back to the peak of coal mining, Appalachia has constantly been embroiled in the contentious jobs-versus-the-environment contest. We often hear that it is possible to have both a clean environment and a thriving economy, but the expectations for and the promises of a thriving economy almost always win when they are competing with environmental protection initiatives. The coal industry offers both historical and contemporary examples of the debate over jobs and the environment. When lawmakers propose regulations calling for stricter controls on coal-fired power plants, we hear how new regulations will cost jobs. For example, a common reaction to the 2015 Clean Power Plan, which focuses on reducing climate-related carbon dioxide emissions, is that the plan will "kill countless jobs in coal and related industries."[17] This is an echo of the billboard rhetoric that decries the War on Coal.

Special interests use opposition to so-called job-killing regulations simultaneously with promises of new jobs in order to support new industries and activities with uncertain environmental health impacts. Drilling for natural gas and oil in Appalachia is a potent example of how people are forced to choose between jobs and the environment. Specifically, the massive incursion of hydraulic fracturing demonstrates that politicians are overplaying the jobs card while minimizing the impact of potential environmental health risks.[18] When the narrative comes across as an ultimatum—choose between jobs and the environment—it is little wonder that economically distressed places end up with a disproportionate number of polluting facilities. This raises the likelihood that there are bona fide pollution havens in Appalachia. A tragedy also emerges, in that generations of families who live in these areas are subject to inequitable exposures because they had no other economic choice.

Pollution Havens in Appalachia

To explore the existence of pollution havens in Appalachia, we must get a sense of how much pollution is released into the environment. The Toxic Release Inventory (TRI) is an important source of local pollution data. The EPA compiles the TRI annually from reports provided by facilities. These reports are required to detail releases (in pounds) of certain chemicals into the air, on the land, in the water, and in underground injection wells. The TRI was enacted in federal legislation after several significant catastrophes, including the 1984 Union Carbide release in Bhopal, India, that killed thousands and left many chronically ill. There was international outrage when it became clear that people living near the plant in Bhopal knew nothing about what they were being exposed to. In the United States, this outrage led to a regulatory approach requiring facilities to report environmental releases so that local people could keep track of chemicals that might make them sick.

Even though the TRI is widely used to compare polluting facilities, for numerous reasons it is a deficient source of pollution information. First, it is based on self-reported data not routinely verified by regulatory agencies. Second, pollutant releases are reported in pounds per year, making visualizing the magnitude of the releases challenging. Finally, data is often reported to the public several years after the releases occur. All these factors affect the reliability of the TRI as a metric for pollution. Regardless, the TRI, though empirically weak, is still one of the best sources of pollution data in the United States at present. Researchers, activists, regulators, and even industry representatives regularly use TRI data to corroborate their arguments. Despite this widespread use, the limitations of the data, specifically when using it to compare places, must be kept in mind.

TRI data indicates that, aside from Texas, Nevada, and Utah, the states within the boundaries of Appalachia document the highest amount of pollution.[19]

Even more alarming is that the risk-screening score, which is an indicator of the health impact from pollution, is higher in some Appalachian states than in states that have higher levels of documented pollution. Within the thirteen Appalachian states, the counties delineated as Appalachia consistently post the highest numbers in the TRI. Some might think that pollution means jobs and that this is evidence that manufacturing and industry are booming. However, when we use the pollution-per-manufacturing-job ratio, evidence emerges that Appalachian counties are possible pollution havens.[20] The average TRI release per manufacturing job in non-Appalachian counties is significantly lower than in Appalachian counties. This means that there is more pollution emitted for every job in Appalachia than for every job outside of the region.

A quantitative analysis using imperfect data does not definitively identify places in Appalachia as pollution havens. However, it does point to exposure inequities in the region. There are significant differences documented between Appalachian and non-Appalachian counties in terms of income, unemployment, health, poverty, and education. Cancer incidence and cancer mortality are also significantly higher in the Appalachian counties. But we cannot draw conclusions about causal relationships between pollution and cancer using secondary data. At the very least, we must continue to question why Appalachian counties with the highest amount of TRI releases are the same counties with the highest cancer rates.

TRI data provide a foundation for applying the pollution-haven hypothesis in Appalachia, but this does not tell the stories about places in the region affected by pollution. There are places in Appalachia that have one industrial facility reporting releases of massive amounts of pollutants. These large facilities produce pollution, not jobs, and share some characteristics with PORTS. People who live in or near these places rely on one facility for their livelihoods. When the industry shuts down, the economic backbone of these places crumbles. This leaves elected officials with few choices to improve economic conditions. In some cases, such as that of Beaver County, Pennsylvania, when another company starts talking about building something new in the area, everyone rolls out the red carpet in welcome, setting up the potential for pollution havens in the future.

The Atomic Effect

The story of the A-Plant in Pike County, Ohio, continues across Appalachia. It was not an unusual case by any means; as a matter of fact, it is typical of how decisions are made in the region. We can look to Beaver County, Pennsylvania, for another example of how communities create pollution havens. This county on the western border of Pennsylvania, along the Ohio River, includes the town of Shippingport, where, in 1958, the first commercial nuclear energy plant was built. This plant was part of a US program known as Atoms for Peace. In the early 1980s it was also the first nuclear energy plant to be decommissioned and decontaminated. Although the Shippingport nuclear power plant was dismantled before we began reporting pollution releases, its legacy contributes to Beaver County being one of the most polluted counties in Pennsylvania.

In 2013, one zinc smelting facility in Beaver County reported more total pollution releases than any other in the state. Until 2014, this location, owned by Horsehead Corporation, employed 510 people. In 2013, the company reported releases of more than 19 million pounds of pollution, or more than 37,000 pounds of pollution for each job at the facility. This one facility not only released the most pollution in the county, it contributed to the fact that Beaver County at this time accounted for almost one-quarter of all TRI releases in the state.[21] In 2014, the company moved its operation to North Carolina and closed the plant in Beaver County, taking its jobs and pollution emissions with it.

The site of the plant would not be empty for long. In July 2015, Shell Chemical of Appalachia, LLC, bought the site of the former smelter. Shell is using the site as part of a strategy to build an ethane cracker plant, calling it the Appalachian Petrochemical Project. A cracker plant takes ethane, which is a by-product of natural gas production, and makes ethylene. Ethylene is used in the production of plastics and other consumer goods. Hydraulic fracturing has increased access to ethane, so cracker plants are being proposed around the country, with several under discussion in Appalachia.

When the Pennsylvania Department of Environmental Protection held a public meeting about the proposed plant, the audience "seemed to warm to the idea of bringing in the plant, citing the economic boost such a project would bring to an area no stranger to industrial development."[22] Another report noted, "officials say 400 to 500 operational jobs and thousands of construction jobs would be created."[23] Beaver County officials were quoted as saying that Shell's plans for the site would be a "game-changer" for the county. They are also portraying a facility that has the potential to bring sixteen to eighteen thousand jobs to the area surrounding the site.[24] However, in 2018, concerns were being raised about the availability of construction workers to build the plant, and workers were being recruited like this: "The short version is this: Unions for carpenters, ironworkers, steamfitters, and heavy equipment operators need more members, more people to help build the facility. Like, now. The unions offer free training. No, the jobs are not permanent, but such jobs never are. They're good, high-paying jobs and the jobs will last at least a few years. Plus you get bragging rights—'I helped build the Shell cracker plant.'"[25]

Sound familiar? Replace "Shell cracker plant" with "Portsmouth Gaseous Diffusion Plant" or "Shippingport Nuclear Power Plant," and nothing has changed in more than sixty years. The Energy Information Administration notes that "ethylene crackers are expensive and complex projects that take many years to develop."[26] So, creating the impression that these plants will dramatically and instantly improve the jobs situation in distressed places is disingenuous at best and deceitful at worst. The planning and permitting phases of these projects could last many months and the construction phase will be short-term, perhaps as little as three years. Once the plant is operational, it could create jobs for as few as 350 people. As the economic prospect for natural gas starts to wane, many facilities tied to drilling, including the one in Beaver County, will generate even fewer jobs than the most conservative estimates. Appalachian places become pollution havens because the people here need jobs and are willing to work hard to support their families. Even knowing that the cracker plant, or the nuclear power plant, or any other potentially hazardous facility will not create long-term employment opportunities does not sway support.

CONNECTING POLLUTION, PLACE, AND HEALTH

Pike County, Ohio, and Beaver County, Pennsylvania, are among the many examples of small places in Appalachia demonstrating the fragile relationship between the economy and environmental health. The measure of pollution per manufacturing job is a simple but illustrative way to gauge the economic impact of some facilities. This indicator is somewhat irrelevant to local people who view any job as a benefit to the community. Nevertheless, because there tend to be larger amounts of pollution per job in Appalachian places than others, it is a starting point for further research and discussion. The TRI figures on releases of pollutants also serve as an imperfect indicator of environmental exposure. This is especially the case with pollution that is reportedly released into the air and water. Pollution does not respect geopolitical boundaries. These releases affect more than just people in the counties in which they are emitted. If there are health impacts related to pollution releases, they are likely to affect multiple counties and places within them.

The connection between exposure to pollution and health outcomes is complicated and difficult to validate. This is especially the case when examining chronic health outcomes, such as cancer, that people tend to associate with environmental exposures. The best that we can do now is to identify locations of pollution sources and locations of cancer cases and examine statistical relationships between the two. It may never be possible to definitively prove that pollution causes cancer, or many other serious health effects, for that matter.

There is plenty of evidence of cancer disparities in Appalachia.[27] Cancer mortality also has been shown to be higher in Appalachia than in the rest of the country and seems to be specifically related to sociodemographic factors such as education and income.[28] As research continues to point to health disparities in the region and environmental exposures are documented to be significantly higher in Appalachia than other places, speculation about the connection between the two will continue. If Appalachian people stand out because they have poor health and Appalachian places stand out because they have poor environments, then pure logic suggests a relationship between the place and health.

6

A Place for Resource Extraction

Anywhere else in this country, when you hear about Appalachia you immediately think, poor people who've been, you know, repeatedly exploited by the lumber industry, the coal mining industry, and left in great poverty, left with the health problems and with the poverty of an industry coming in, taking the resources and leaving. And so it's just odd to me that Appalachia doesn't remember what's been done and repeated promises. And then look at where we are, after all those wave after wave of [exploitive] industries, who've come through here taking the resources and leaving the mess and leaving. And so I just, I don't know, how do we get people to remember?

—Resident of Appalachia, returning from Colorado

Coal mining and fracking are severely deteriorating the environment in the region.

—Appalachian environmental health professional

JUST HEARING THE WORD APPALACHIA CONJURES IMAGES OF mountains and rural areas brimming with natural resources. Appalachia has been described as "a rich land inhabited by a poor people."[1] The wealth of the land is found in its energy-producing resources like timber, coal, and natural gas. Most of Appalachia is in the broad physiographic region known as the

Appalachian Highlands and is subdivided into the Appalachian Plateau, Blue Ridge, and Valley and Ridge subregions. The Appalachian Plateau subregion comprises the largest portion of Appalachia and most of the natural resources that are the source of economic growth are here.

The drive into the Appalachian Plateau from Ohio to southwest Virginia follows Route 23 south the entire way. As you leave southern Ohio and cross into Kentucky, the rolling hills of Appalachia become more substantial, and as you enter Virginia from Kentucky, the hills transform into legitimate mountains. This route winds through many small towns that begin to look the same after several hours, seemingly each with its Walmart, several McDonalds, a Taco Bell, and the Dollar General. There are also boarded-up businesses, ample properties for sale or lease, and train tracks crisscrossing the entire route. It is not necessary to travel far from the main highway to find other similarities that are less obvious but more relevant to environmental health in Appalachia. The coalfields or company towns nestled in the mountains serve as remnants of the influence of coal on the region.

In the case of Virginia, coal was discovered in the southwestern part of the state in the late 1800s, but it wasn't until the railroad extended into the region that the fate of this place was sealed. Trains moved coal out of the area, but they were not used for moving workers into it. Coal companies created small towns to ensure workers remained close to the mines. Life in the coal camps was unjust and harsh, especially considering the occupational dangers of underground mining. The injustice continued after the mines closed and the workers left the camps. When coal companies were done with a mine, they would sell or abandon houses and walk away from the camps, leaving remaining residents exposed to existing and emergent environmental problems. Picture a cluster of houses constructed quickly and shoddily, without access to drinking-water and wastewater infrastructure, and one can imagine a range of environmental health issues in these company towns.

On April 15, 1915, a front-page article in the *Big Stone Gap (Virginia) Post*, quoting the state Board of Health about controlling typhoid, told this story: "An insanitary town has a bad name. This reacts on its trade and its development as well as on the health of its people. On the other hand, the small towns which have a good water supply and a sewerage system or a well-enforced sanitary privy ordinance are almost certain to attract settlers."[2]

Imboden is a coal company town built in 1902 in Wise County, Virginia, near the towns of Big Stone Gap and Appalachia. John Imboden was a Civil

War general, a Virginia state legislator, and the owner of one of the first coal companies in the state. The unincorporated community is located on a strip of flat land between a small creek and a mountain. A railroad track separates the homes from the creek and runs parallel to it for many miles. For decades, sewage from the town's fourteen houses flowed through straight pipes discharging high levels of bacteria and other contaminants directly into the creek. As late as the 1980s, there were as many as twenty thousand straight pipes in southwest Virginia, contributing to significant environmental and public health concerns.[3] Appalachian coal camps and company towns are prime locations for straight-pipe sewage and consequential sources of water contamination. The geography and topography of these places create serious challenges in installing systems for water management. In the early 1990s, wastewater treatment technologies emerged that could handle low flows from individual properties and small communities. These advances in treatment options can address the environmental health problems with raw sewage, and Imboden provides one example of success.

In 1998, Imboden residents collaborated with public health officials to initiate the Imboden Community Wastewater Treatment Project. The mission of the project was to tackle the legacy of sewage contaminating nearby waterways for decades. With funding from multiple sources, including the Tennessee Valley Authority, the National Small Flows Clearinghouse, and individual homeowners, the community is now equipped with wastewater treatment that includes shared septic tanks and a sewage collection system. Operating and maintaining wastewater treatment facilities can be more expensive than constructing them, so Imboden partners with the nearby town of Appalachia for some of these services.

Driving through the coalfields of southwestern Virginia today, it is obvious that Imboden is different than some of the other towns nearby. The houses appear to be maintained better, people seem a little more welcoming, and this place looks more like a neighborhood than a cluster of run-down houses. There is even hope that the wastewater improvements could contribute to Imboden being designated as a national historical landmark.[4] There is no doubt that eliminating straight piping of sewage has improved environmental conditions. Environmental monitoring shows significant reductions in levels of nitrogen, E. coli, and other contaminants entering the creek.[5] So, more than a hundred years after the Board of Health noted the importance of clean water for community health and prosperity, conditions in Imboden are finally improving.

What remains to be seen is whether cases such as the Imboden success story can make a dent in the severe economic conditions in Wise County, which posts some of the highest unemployment and poverty rates in the state. Improving conditions in local places, such as coal camps like Imboden, contribute to the environment vs. economy conundrum, for improvements in environmental and public health do not necessarily lead to better economic health. The Imboden story also highlights the complicated relationship that Appalachian places have with coal. Residents view coal as both beneficial and wicked, but even those who are alarmed about the health and environmental impacts of coal understand its historical importance in the economy of local places. The population in Wise County is dwindling and Big Stone Gap is trying to redefine itself as a tourist destination, but everyone I spoke to near Imboden blames the current economic problems in the area on the decline of coal.

As environmental health scenarios play out with coal mining, hydraulic fracturing (fracking) is emerging, with familiar promises of creating thousands of jobs while contributing to the nation's energy independence. The arguments in favor of coal mining are being replayed throughout Appalachia as fracking invades the region with its temporary economic benefits and little evidence of consideration for long-term environmental and health consequences. Meanwhile, the public health effects of coal mining are still surfacing, ranging from chronic conditions suffered by individual miners to water quality issues affecting entire communities. Appalachia's experiences with the latent environmental and public health impacts of coal should serve as a warning. It might be best to be cautious about sacrificing natural resources today without clearly understanding effects on the future of the land and its people. This is a warning those pushing for increased fracking would be wise to heed, so that shale gas does not become the twenty-first-century coal.

BOOM, BUST, AND HEALTH: ACT I

Imboden is just one of many coal company towns dotted throughout Appalachia amidst a backdrop of one of the most beautiful places in the country. Coal has been the foundation of the rural Appalachian economy for more than a hundred years. Its life cycle from mining to burning contributes to long-term environmental contamination and affects public health in ways that are still emerging today.

At first, coal was abundant and easy to mine. It was the source of a considerable number of jobs and there was little thought to its sustainability. How could, and why should, people with an immediate need to earn a living worry about potential future economic, environmental, and public health consequences? Now, we look at coal in the early twenty-first century and we see that, as its economic influence blackens, its environmental health impacts deepen. Mining jobs are dissipating like morning fog over the Appalachian Mountains, while mountaintop removal is irreparably changing the environment and catastrophic accidents involving mining wastes are wreaking havoc on small communities. At the same time, miners are being killed and injured in accidents that are preventable if minimal safety protocols are followed. Even in this context, many politicians and residents from Appalachian coal mining states remain steadfast in their support for the industry. They hunger for a return of boom times, a return that will never happen.

Take a close look at the history of coal mining and what you see are boom-and-bust cycles in which there are spurts of new jobs followed by periods of record-high unemployment. Many accounts of coal mining in Appalachia highlight the effect of the industry's instability on the region's people and environment.[6] While the history of Appalachian coal draws attention to the importance of the place in meeting national priorities, Appalachia remains a vital study in assessing and understanding the impact of coal in the United States. One indicator of this is what is known as the Central Appalachian (CAPP) delivery zone, which is a distribution hub for coal from the region. The CAPP includes portions of southeastern Ohio, northeastern Kentucky, and western West Virginia. The US Energy Information Administration uses the CAPP as a benchmark for monitoring prices for all coal that is mined in the eastern part of the country.[7]

Even though more than 80 percent of the underground and surface coal mines in the United States are in Appalachia, coal's tenuous position as a driver of the Appalachian economy is becoming clearer every year.[8] There are many reasons for coal's decline, including innovations in mining technology, increases in extraction and transportation costs, new regulations, a push for more efficient and sustainable energy sources, the overall state of the economy, and the availability of natural gas and oil.[9] These factors, combined with a weakening domestic demand for coal, have precipitated economic effects which are rippling throughout Appalachian communities. With the steady reduction in the demand for coal and therefore mining, it might seem reasonable to see a decline in the public health consequences of coal as well. Not so; in fact, both occupational and environmental health impacts continue to proliferate.

The Health of Miners

Historically, the influence of Appalachian coal on the economy extended well beyond the coalfields of the region, as it was a critical driver of the industrial revolution.[10] While the economic benefits of coal mined in Appalachia were reaped across the country and the world, the nation's prosperity came at the expense of public health near the mines. Mining, transporting, and burning coal contribute to health outcomes in diverse and deleterious ways. In the early days of mining and for many decades, the health of coal miners was of little concern to anyone but the miners and their families. For more than a hundred years, miners were exposed to both catastrophic and prolonged adverse conditions, leading to acute and chronic health outcomes. Injuries and deaths from unsafe mines and illnesses such as chronic respiratory conditions were common, but it was rare for mining companies to be held accountable. The lack of accountability for unsafe conditions was the main reason that miners unionized in the late 1800s, resulting in historic clashes between miners and mine owners. The mine workers' unions held mine owners accountable for the hazardous conditions in the mines.

The federal government did not get involved in general occupational safety and health until the late 1960s. In response to public outcry over dangerous working conditions across the country, Congress ratified the Occupational Safety and Health Act in 1970. This law established the Occupational Safety and Health Administration (OSHA), which is responsible for writing and enforcing federal standards targeting workplace safety. OSHA focuses on multiple workplaces, not just mines. It would be several years after its founding before governmental oversight of mine safety was institutionalized. The Mine Safety and Health Administration (MSHA) was established in 1978. The Mine Safety and Health Act of 1977 mandated protection of both the rights and the health of miners. All this federal institution-building and law-making was critical to making mining safer, but it was a hundred years too late for more than a generation of miners.

Today, the Centers for Disease Control and Prevention's National Institute of Occupational Safety and Health (NIOSH) oversees health screening of coal miners in compliance with rules from the MSHA. NIOSH coordinates the Coal Workers' Health Surveillance Program, which offers medical testing to miners.

Until 2014, only underground miners were included in the program, but the surveillance program now includes all miners, so surface miners are eligible to participate. In addition, the 2014 rules pertaining to miners' occupational exposures were revised for the purpose of strengthening protective measures to reduce respiratory disease among miners.[11] The revised rules offer all miners the right to participate in free respiratory health screenings, including chest x-rays and lung-function tests.

Chronic conditions such as coal workers' pneumoconiosis (CWP, or black lung disease), silicosis, and chronic obstructive pulmonary disease (COPD) are increasing. Specifically, black lung disease, which results from inhaling mine dust, is seeing a resurgence in Appalachia.[12] This is especially troubling because more younger miners are suffering now. Occupational exposures are intensifying as underground coal becomes more inaccessible, causing miners to go deeper into less ventilated spaces.[13] Those who are mining above ground are also being diagnosed with preventable respiratory illnesses. The CDC reports that the prevalence of mining-related illnesses is higher in Central Appalachia than other US mining regions.[14]

Even if miners do not have a preventable respiratory disease, they work in one of the most dangerous occupations in the country. MHSA posts accounts of annual fatalities related to coal mining, and every year about twenty US miners die on the job. Tragically, some catastrophes result in multiple deaths. One such accident occurred in April 2010, when twenty-nine miners were killed in an explosion at the Upper Big Branch Mine in Montcoal, West Virginia. This is still one of the largest coal mining disasters in the United States. MSHA's investigation concluded that it could have been prevented if the mine owners and managers had complied with regulations.[15] In investigating the Upper Big Branch explosion, MSHA found that Performance Coal Company and Massey Energy (PCC/Massey) created a culture of profit over safety and took little interest in training miners or ensuring that devices to monitor explosive gases were in working condition. MSHA identified many flagrant violations, including PCC/Massey's deliberate and intentional cover-up of hazardous conditions to keep them hidden from mine inspectors.

In the eighteen months prior to the explosion at Upper Big Branch, MSHA inspectors identified 684 violations at the mine and proposed more than $1.3 million dollars in penalties. Of the 684 violations, 56 "were the result of the Operator's unwarrantable failure to comply with mandatory safety and health standards."[16] So how was this mine able to keep operating, considering that its owners were flagrantly violating the law? Some argue that the law is weak, and fines are ineffective since unpaid penalties do not shut down mines. Perhaps weak enforcement of mine safety laws and regulations is because of the lack of available resources; enforcing regulations are only as strong as the budget allows. In fact, MSHA's internal review determined that resource constraints were an underlying factor in the Upper Big Branch tragedy. Regardless of the myriad failures on the part of the industry and government, Appalachia consistently accounts for more than its share of fatalities associated with coal mining. West Virginia is the deadliest state, posting 123 fatalities since 2005.[17]

Mining Places

While occupational health is an essential component of public health, coal miners are a relatively narrow population. Beyond miners, there are more broadly reaching environmental public health effects from coal mining that are exceedingly well documented in Appalachia. For example, living near a mining operation, in particular a mountaintop-removal site, is associated with numerous ailments, including serious respiratory conditions and cancers as well as poor health-related quality of life.[18] Coal's lifecycle creates place-based public health issues that start from mining and continue through transporting and burning coal. The environmental public health effects are just as chronic as the respiratory diseases suffered by miners, because they continue for decades on wasted landscapes and in polluted waters.

Company towns such as Imboden are part of coal's lifecycle and are places in which public health is directly and indirectly affected by mining. These environmental health impacts are expansive, and as long as consumers flip switches for lights, appliances, and devices, they will continue. The company town is near the mine, but once mined, coal often travels long distances to distribution hubs or power plants. Throughout the Appalachian coalfields, there are railroad tracks running parallel to waterways, from small creeks to major rivers. Coal accounts for a large percentage of the commodity rail transport in the United States, most of it coming from western states.[19] Western coal, with its lower sulfur content, is more attractive than Appalachian coal because it saves money in complying with air pollution regulations. This means that coal is moving around the country on long, slow-moving trains for hundreds of miles.

West Virginia ranks second for the amount of coal that is loaded onto trains and moved around the country. You are likely to see coal trains moving through the Appalachian states of Kentucky, Pennsylvania, Virginia, and Ohio as well.

Even though coal transport in West Virginia comprises only a small percentage of all the coal shipped by rail nationwide, coal trains account for almost 100 percent of rail cargo originating in the state and for a significant portion of the end of the line for trains. To put this more simply, almost every freight rail car traveling in and through West Virginia contains coal either coming into or leaving the state.

Considering the volume of coal transported by rail, accidents are rare events that primarily lead to economic losses to the railroad. However, sometimes a derailment creates a public health threat. In December 2014, a train carrying coal through Paris, Kentucky, derailed, dumping some of its load into a creek. The hazards of this derailment were compounded because it not only contaminated the creek with coal, it also damaged a sewage line, spilling wastewater into the creek along with the coal.

Once coal reaches its destination, it might be burned to produce energy for people who live hundreds of miles away. The local and global environmental health effects from coal-fired power plants are well-understood and documented. Burning high-sulfur coal from Appalachia creates sulfur dioxide and nitrogen dioxide. These two pollutants must be monitored and managed to comply with regulations from the Clean Air Act (CAA). The CAA establishes National Ambient Air Quality Standards (NAAQS), which, while national in scope, are mostly enforced by state and local governments. Every state must monitor pollutant levels and develop plans for EPA approval to address places that fail to meet the NAAQS.

Sulfur dioxide is a major air pollutant from burning coal and has local and regional environmental health impacts. Southeastern Ohio, western Pennsylvania, including Beaver County, and two counties in West Virginia do not meet national standards for sulfur dioxide. That is, these places are "nonattainment" areas for complying with the regulations.[20] The nonattainment areas are in rural Appalachian places that emit high amounts of pollutants because of large facilities. When people are exposed to high levels of sulfur dioxide for short periods of time, it can feel like their airways are burning. High-level exposures typically result from accidents rather than the day-to-day pollution that comes out of smokestacks at power plants. Lingering health effects tied to these chronic exposures include changes in lung function and increased incidence of asthma.

Oxides of nitrogen are another group of pollutants that form when coal is burned. The health effects of exposure to nitrogen oxides are like those associated with sulfur dioxide. Short-term exposures to high levels make it difficult to breathe and aggravate asthma. Long-term exposures can cause asthma or respiratory infections. One notable difference between sulfur and nitrogen pollution from coal burning is that nitrogen oxides can combine with other chemicals in the air to create ozone and particulate matter, two components of smog. Sulfur and nitrogen in the forms they are released from power plants also contribute to acid rain, an important concern threatening ecosystem health, especially in the northeastern United States.

Let's turn our attention to a notorious situation in an Appalachian Ohio place where the community health impacts of coal have been extensively documented. Cheshire, Ohio, in Gallia County, abuts the Ohio River, where coal barges float all day. The focal point of Cheshire is the General James M. Gavin Power Plant, the largest coal-fired power plant in Ohio when measured by the amount of electricity it generates. Gavin relies on high-sulfur Appalachian coal, and this has created the need for air pollution control equipment to meet emission limits in the plant's operating permit. Even though Gavin is generally in compliance with regulations, it still releases a large quantity of air pollutants. The Gavin Power Plant is one reason why Ohio tends to rank in the top ten in the country for overall emissions, as reported in the Toxic Release Inventory.

In the late 1990s, Gavin was exceeding the emissions of nitrogen dioxide allowed in its permit. As a result, the plant owner, American Electric Power (AEP), installed pollution control equipment known as the selective catalytic reduction (SCR) system. The SCR system introduces ammonia into the smokestack to reduce emissions of nitrogen oxides. After the SCR system was installed in 2001, sulfur emissions, in the form of sulfuric acid, almost doubled in just one year.[21] As these emissions increased, Cheshire residents were subject to acute air pollution events referred to as plume touchdowns. When weather conditions were right, a cloud of air pollutants would veer to the ground in people's backyards. Since the plumes contained sulfuric acid, nitrogen oxides, and other pollutants, residents suffered acute health effects such as sore throats, eye irritation, and trouble breathing. AEP and the Ohio EPA monitored air quality in Cheshire and measured extremely high levels of sulfuric acid in the local environment. They found that installing equipment to solve one pollution problem had created another.

Faced with the potential for litigation related to health claims, combined with the corporate economic consequences of failing to rapidly solve the sulfuric acid problem, AEP proposed a plan to directly compensate residents. This plan included negotiating with interested property owners to purchase their homes. Those who agreed to the terms of sale would not be able to sue AEP for future health outcomes. Once implemented, AEP purchased the entire village for twenty million dollars. Some people chose not to sell and remain in the village, and today about 132 people, or about one-half of the population prior to the buyout, still live near the Gavin plant.

The Cheshire Transaction, as it became known, sparked debate both inside and outside of the community. Inside the village there was tension between neighbors, while those outside village boundaries argued about the ethics of being excluded from the negotiation. In the end, Cheshire as a place was altered forever due to public health concerns regarding this step in coal's lifecycle and serves as a powerful example of the complexities of environmental health in a region in which the coal industry dominates. Cheshire and Imboden illustrate how coal generates short-term economic benefits while creating long-term, place-based public and environmental health effects. These effects continue long after the mining, transporting, and burning of coal stops. These communities and many others might predict the future of Appalachia's role in the next energy boom: natural gas.

BOOM, BUST, AND HEALTH: ACT II

Consider the following passage from a 1990 report: "Burial of waste is accompanied by isolation practices, whereby the wastes are encapsulated in clay materials that are designed to minimize leakage or leaching of toxic materials. Care is taken to avoid placement of wastes in areas where a high contamination potential exists. However, little is known about the long-term effects of such burial practices on the quality of recharge to groundwater."[22]

The uncertainty noted in this passage is from a report about the potential environmental effects of surface mining for coal. However, the same uncertainties exist today with natural gas and oil, and we can replace "coal mining" with "hydraulic fracturing" in studies and reports written decades ago. Although natural gas and oil are historical components of Appalachia's energy portfolio, tremendous increases in drilling activity are creating new boom conditions in many local places. The geology of Appalachia has once again put the region at the center of efforts to provide a resource that will benefit not only the United States, but other nations as well. One author writing about natural gas notes, "This once quiet stepchild fuel raised in the hills of Appalachia now must reconcile the hopes and fears of a nation."[23]

For decades, drilling for natural gas and oil mostly involved vertical wells, a process that constrains production to relatively small areas. When the first horizontal well was attempted in 1929 in Texas, it was clear that turning the drill bit at the bottom of a vertical well would expand production and minimize costs. To further enhance well production, the unconventional method of hydraulic fracturing (fracking) was used with vertical oil wells as early as 1947, but only recently has fracking been combined with horizontal drilling as a means of further enhancing well productivity.[24] Now the term fracking is used to describe a process involving extensive site preparation, drilling vertically and horizontally, using large quantities of water, injecting chemicals into the well, and generating significant amounts of liquid waste.

Fracking and Health

In the United States, current regulatory approaches to fracking are inconsistent because individual states are responsible for overseeing the process. State legislatures are making policy decisions about fracking in the context of little credible and peer-reviewed research related to the immediate and long-term environmental health consequences. Understanding the environmental health impacts of fracking is complicated by public opinion, which is being driven by messages both in favor of and opposed to the process. In addition, the boom in fracking occurred against a backdrop of general concern about the economy and public opinion polls showing Americans more concerned about the state of the economy than many other issues.[25]

Once again, the economy in Appalachia plays a significant role in the lack of precaution in natural resource extraction. We can see this in the dash to drill without scientific studies addressing its health and environmental impacts. New York is one of a few states that took a precautionary approach when the governor banned hydraulic fracturing in 2015. His decision was based on advice from state public health and environmental officials. Meanwhile, several Appalachian states, including Pennsylvania, Ohio, Kentucky, and West Virginia, proceeded with rapid and almost uncontrolled drilling.

Scientists are sprinting to catch up with drillers to build a cache of data that might be useful to decision makers and public health officials. Most of the fracking research to date is focusing on environmental monitoring rather than environmental health. This monitoring research measures levels of pollutants in groundwater or air that can be specifically linked to fracking. Many of these studies have been prompted by citizen concerns about the possible health consequences of living near fracking activities. While the EPA has found contaminants in drinking water, the agency is not ready to say that fracking is causing the contamination, even if it agrees there are public health risks.

In 2009, the EPA tested two municipal wells and thirty-seven residential wells in Pavillion, Wyoming; about one year later, they tested three shallow monitoring wells and forty-one private wells. Based on the monitoring data, federal public health officials recommended an alternate source of water for private-well users. The recommendation took into consideration a range of contaminants, including those associated with natural gas production and those that are naturally occurring, such as arsenic and sodium. In 2011, the EPA tested additional wells in Pavillion. The public was invited to comment on a draft report from this testing until September 2013.[26] However, in June 2013, the EPA issued a statement that it would not seek peer review or finalize the draft, "nor does the agency plan to rely upon the conclusions in the draft report."[27] The Wyoming Department of Environmental Quality continued to study the situation, releasing a draft report in late 2015. The EPA commented on the report, noting that there should be more discussion of the uncertainties when it comes to quantifying health impacts from the contaminants found in the monitoring wells.

Pavillion, Wyoming, laid the foundation for the EPA's approach to other sites, including those in Appalachia. In 2010, the Pennsylvania Department of Environmental Protection sent data to the EPA about environmental contaminants in eighteen wells in the town of Dimock. Testing indicated higher-than-expected levels of methane and organic chemicals specifically associated with natural gas development. The EPA issued a "do not use until further notice" recommendation for the sampled wells. This recommendation was tempered with statements about uncertainty regarding the sampling methodology, since a contractor gathered the data. In 2012, EPA scientists went to Dimock and tested sixty-four wells. Although they found measurable levels of methane and organic chemicals, they concluded that the levels recorded did not pose a public health risk. As the EPA was packing up tits testing kits, local officials lifted the boil order and told residents they could begin using their wells again.

While the EPA was working on understanding potential drinking-water impacts, Congress directed the Government Accountability Office (GAO) to provide information about the potential for natural gas production from shale and the environmental and public health risks associated with hydraulic fracturing. Sometimes referred to as the congressional watchdog, the GAO is an independent, nonpartisan agency that works for Congress. To answer the questions about possible health risks, GAO staff reviewed "more than 90 studies and other publications from federal agencies and laboratories, state agencies, local governments, the petroleum industry, academic institutions, environmental and public health groups, and other nongovernmental organizations." Few of these studies were in peer-reviewed journals; rather, they were government reports and articles in professional journals. The GAO published its report in 2012 concluding, "the risks identified in the studies and publications we reviewed cannot, at present, be quantified, and the magnitude of potential adverse effects or the likelihood of occurrence cannot be determined."[28]

To further emphasize the inconclusiveness and uncertainty around the science related to environmental and public health risks of fracking, the Research Triangle Environmental Health Collaborative organized a summit in October 2012.[29] This collaborative is a nonprofit organization focusing on research and discourse related to important environmental health issues. The 2012 summit involved three workgroups to discuss human exposures, social impacts, and health impact assessments. The proceedings from the summit identify numerous uncertainties in understanding the range of impacts from shale gas development.[30] Among these uncertainties are the lack of background data on the current state of groundwater in areas ripe for fracking, the possible impacts to vulnerable populations, and the chemical and nonchemical risks to ecosystems.

The 2012 summit also identified issues with emergency preparedness to address the range of possible accidents during the fracking process. There has been little discussion of worst-case scenarios with fracking, even though responses to other energy-related accidents document widespread environmental health repercussions directly related to poor planning. For example, using the 2010 Deepwater Horizon oil spill in the Gulf of Mexico as an example for preparing for fracking accidents, the uncoordinated and weak response highlighted the need for regulators to "understand technologies that have potential devastating environmental consequences if things go awry and regulate commensurate with the level of risk presented to minimize threats to human health and the environment."[31] Unfortunately, it is likely to take a major accident at a fracking site, a ruptured pipeline that affects a large area, or some other catastrophe to draw attention to the potential hazards of the fracking process.

Scientists conducting environmental monitoring found chemicals in drinking-water wells, but as we entered the 2010s there was still little data to support drawing conclusions about what the public health impacts could be. This led the EPA to plan a comprehensive approach to gathering data about the drinking-water impacts of fracking. Agency scientists reviewed existing studies, examined retrospective case studies, applied various computer models to evaluate different scenarios, and conducted laboratory and toxicological investigations. Even after looking at about twelve hundred sources of data and gathering input from stakeholders, the EPA was unable to make a definitive statement about the drinking-water impacts from fracking. The final report identifies numerous ways in which fracking could affect drinking water, including interfering with water quality and contaminating groundwater during a spill or injection of waste.

While the report agrees that there are potential impacts, it also states that "it was not possible to fully characterize the severity of impacts, nor was it possible to calculate or estimate the national frequency of impacts."[32] So, the EPA's years-long comprehensive study clearly indicates a range of uncertainties in understanding the environmental health impacts of fracking. In addition, the study was completed almost twenty years after fracking began booming. Those places that welcomed fracking as a cure-all to their economic woes did so without regard to environmental and public health.

While the EPA was conducting its study, the agency hosted activities to keep people informed of their work. During a webinar early on, the EPA reported some of the results of five retrospective case studies, two of which were in Appalachia. The case studies suggested the presence of methane in drinking-water wells, but the lead researcher explained that it is impossible to say that fracking caused the contamination. The ambiguity about the effects of fracking on drinking water is the result of a lack of historical groundwater data in general. A significant portion of the groundwater in the United States is used by homeowners through private wells, which are typically not monitored or regulated by state or local health officials. These wells are not routinely tested for contamination.

Determining the link between environmental conditions and public health outcomes is a daunting task. Researchers have a long way to go to produce a body of scientific evidence that offers credible and peer-reviewed information about the relationship between fracking and public health. It will take many years and many more analyses to scientifically answer so many questions about how people and places could be affected both now and in the future. The lack of peer-reviewed research on the consequences of fracking contributes to both proponents and opponents using what little is available to support their contradictory views. The lack of science means that policy is likely to be driven more by public opinion than empirical evidence, and public opinion is related to how the existing science is portrayed by those actively engaged in the fracking debate. Except in New York, as noted above, scientific uncertainty has done little to slow fracking in Appalachia.

The Place of Fracking

As was the case with coal mining in the nineteenth and twentieth centuries, the natural resources of Appalachia have again combined with economic imperatives, creating an opportune time for fracking to thrive. From 2000 through 2009, the United States experienced two recessions. The first one began in March 2001 and ended in November 2001, when the economy contracted to its lowest point.[33] The second began in December 2007 and continued until June 2009, making it the longest recession since World War II.[34] Between 2000 and 2009, the number of producing natural gas wells in the United States rose 30 percent.[35] Wells producing gas in four Appalachian states (West Virginia, Ohio, Kentucky, and Pennsylvania) rose by 21 percent from 2000 to 2009. So, as natural gas production was increasing rapidly, the country experienced two recessions—an important point, since those who argue in favor of fracking contend that it will solve economic problems.

Flash forward to the 2010s, and the advanced technology enabling fracking has created conditions in local places that can be compared to those from coal mining in the late 1800s. Carroll County, Ohio, offers a prime example of the positive and negative effects of the fracking boom. Located in the northeastern corner of the state on the western edge of Appalachia, the county has no four-lane roads. It is common to get stuck behind large farm equipment, since agriculture has been the predominant local economic activity for decades. The county exemplifies the meaning of the word "bucolic," with the rolling hills that define Appalachian Ohio. Dotted throughout these rolling hills are hundreds of active oil and gas wells drilled using the hydraulic fracturing technique.[36]

When I visited Carroll County in the summer of 2013, the impact of the shale gas boom was apparent. Slow-moving farm equipment had been replaced with trucks hauling water, chemicals, and brine to and from well pads. New roads had been built, and signs posted on some of the old unmarked gravel roads warned truck drivers from the drilling company to keep out. According to one local official, the main drilling company in the county had spent more than $40 million on road infrastructure since drilling began—compared to the annual county road improvement budget of $600,000.

All the land in Carroll County that is likely to be used by energy companies for fracking has already been leased, and one estimate suggests that 95 percent of the mineral rights in the county are now in the hands of oil and gas companies.[37] The leases and purchases mainly benefit private landowners, who negotiate with the energy companies for a price per acre. Even with the additional money, people are not making major purchases; many farmers are paying off their debt and reinvesting in their farms.[38] Local sales tax revenues have increased from truck sales and hotel reservations, and there are indirect benefits to some businesses from home improvements being made by residents. Some people are also optimistic about the impact that fracking will have on the school district, which hasn't passed a levy for capital improvements since the early 1970s.

Looking more closely at the impacts of fracking in Carroll County, it becomes clear that local people have not benefited from the jobs associated with drilling activity, unless they are truck drivers. The roughnecks who work on the drilling rigs are mostly transient, moving from place to place with the drilling companies. Instead of creating company towns for what will be a short-term job, the energy companies put the workers up in the hotels that started popping out of the earth like crocuses in the spring. Like spring crocuses, the profitability of and need for these hotels is short-lived.

There is occasional friction between roughnecks and locals, and calls to the sheriff have doubled in recent years. Another problem with the pace of drilling in the county is that drilling rigs do not have specific addresses. This makes it difficult for first responders to locate accidents, like the one in February 2014, when a worker was killed on a rig site. All in all, local government services such as the health department, law enforcement, and environmental services face significant challenges dealing with the new demands from drilling activities.

The Carroll County situation offers a caution to places that are willing to become inundated with fracking to improve their economic conditions. As a 2014 impact assessment put it, "Communities also face great costs to increase training, road maintenance, police, fire, and other government infrastructure. At the same time, industry development has increased local tax revenue, helping schools and communities in an economically distressed region that has suffered from declining state contributions to schools and local government. In short, the development has fallen far short of expectations, and caused environmental, housing, infrastructure and health problems."[39]

As with coal exploitation, one of the main arguments offered in favor of fracking was that it would create desperately needed jobs. In 2011, when Ohio public officials spoke of the economic impact from shale, they argued that it would attract more than two hundred thousand jobs to the state.[40] As of June 2013, the number of new jobs specifically linked to shale exploration was "disappointing."[41] In her executive summary, the author of the 2014 impact assessment notes that "jobs have been added in Carroll County, but far fewer than promised."[42] The state job market has fluctuated over the years, and 2017 estimates from the Ohio Department of Job and Family Services indicate that there were a little more than sixteen thousand jobs in "core shale-related industry."[43]

Of course, any job estimates do not consider the ripple effects of the industry in small communities. Restaurants get busy, hotels fill up, and stores see sales grow because workers need goods and services. There is also ancillary shale-related employment that includes everything from water suppliers to environmental consultants. The number of jobs related to these ancillary services has grown, but data from the federal government do not specifically link any of the jobs to shale gas. It is an exercise in smoke and mirrors to use the promise of jobs to promote fracking, especially since many of the jobs are temporary and, once wells are in production, the need for workers decreases dramatically. In the case of the counties in Appalachian Ohio where fracking is rampant, unemployment remains higher than the state average, so out-of-state workers may be benefitting more than the local workforce.[44]

For local economies, the sustainability of fracking is dubious. Gas and oil are nonrenewable resources, which, like coal, will inevitably be depleted. There are documented increases in local tax revenues, some businesses are improving their bottom lines, and individual landowners are reaping the benefits from leases and royalties. However, the acute strain on housing in many of the most active drilling counties suggests that these economic gains are not likely improving much-needed employment opportunities for local people.

When coal mining began in the United States, there was no evidence of long-term environmental ramifications, but today, many Appalachian communities are paying for yesterday's quest for cheap energy. Without rational and long-range economic planning, there is a real risk that the shale gas drilling boom will eventually result in a bust not unlike the one that has become the legacy of coal. A few decades from now, Appalachian places may be once again faced with health-threatening environmental conditions resulting from the rush by outsiders to extract the region's natural resources.

Numerous uncertainties exist about the risks of horizontal hydraulic fracturing, but in the context of environmental justice, the question of sustainability is critical. When we made decisions about coal mining so many years ago, the concept of sustainability was not part of the public vernacular. Coal mines seemed like bottomless pits of energy resources, and it was unthinkable that we might one day need an alternative. Today, sustainability is viewed as comprising three spheres: economy, environment, and society. When we use sustainability to guide environmental policy, we are also addressing environmental justice. From this perspective, fracking in Appalachia has the potential to add to the burdens that are at the heart of environmental injustice and inequities in the region.

Coal mining left a legacy of environmental destruction in Appalachia consisting of severe wastewater contamination, deforested hillsides, abandoned mines, acid mine drainage, and piles of waste that dot the landscape. The environmental health impacts of coal are still emerging in the region even though the coal industry is declining. Coal has contributed directly and indirectly to health disparities in Appalachia. When it comes to fracking, one of the major concerns is the potential groundwater contamination from both drilling and waste disposal. Like coal mining in the early 1900s, fracking is proceeding rapidly and, in the absence of evidence from scientific studies, "nearly everyone who draws water from an aquifer above or in the vicinity of fracking activity is a guinea pig."[45]

Perhaps it is the social sphere of sustainability that highlights the environmental inequities of natural resource use in Appalachia. Like coal mining, fracking is concentrated in rural Appalachian counties where the geology supports oil and natural gas deposits. Appalachian people already suffer from health disparities related to behaviors, poverty, education, and health care access. There are multiple policy challenges related to fracking, but we need these policies to address sustainability and the economic, environmental, and social impacts of hydraulic fracturing. Without attention to the disproportionate and inequitable effects of fracking, it can worsen health disparities linked to the environment throughout rural America, repeating a cycle that Appalachia's residents know all too well.

7

A Place for Disasters

And the floods, even though they're very destructive and changed [the village] considerably, because FEMA came through and bought out a bunch of houses . . . the floods were very destructive from that perspective, but the floods really drew the community together.

—Twenty-five-year resident of Appalachia, Ohio

West Virginians do not believe in climate change, and no scientist is going to convince the masses.

—Appalachian environmental health professional

IN WINTER 2008, A BARRIER AROUND A POND HOLDING COAL ash ruptured and the sludge-like water spewed forth in Appalachian Tennessee. More than five million cubic yards, or almost 1.1 billion gallons, of contaminated sludge gushed from the retention pond at the Kingston Fossil Plant. The sludge eventually covered about three hundred acres of land and contaminated two rivers, a reservoir, and soil above private drinking-water wells. This is the largest coal-ash spill in US history. Leaking coal-ash impoundments are human-made, or unnatural, environmental disasters that afflict Appalachian places and can affect public health.

In spring 2011, severe storms with tornadoes and heavy rainfall swept through Appalachia. The Federal Emergency Management Agency (FEMA) declared nine major disasters during a ten-day period in six Appalachian states. Throughout the region, several areas set records for rainfall as measured by the National Oceanic and Atmospheric Administration (NOAA).[1] Southeastern Ohio, western Pennsylvania, northwestern West Virginia, and northern and southeastern Kentucky received more than three times the normal spring rainfall. NOAA ranked the flooding fourth on their list of the top ten national weather/climate events in 2011. Seven years later, Tennessee, North Carolina, Virginia, West Virginia, Pennsylvania, and Maryland would break records for rainfall and 2018 became the wettest year ever.[2]

Whether natural or unnatural in origin, floods cause significant economic, health, and environmental impacts every year. They are the most persistent and costly natural disasters and Appalachian places deal with them almost continuously. Examining the history of staggering disasters in Appalachia provides a warning for the future because of the region's geography, economy, and bureaucracy. When faced with some of the largest floods on record or with historic human-made industrial disasters, Appalachian people have suffered hardship and demonstrated resilience. Overall, disasters in the region highlight the strengths and weaknesses in the capacity of communities to respond to extreme events and point to environmental inequities that underly many of the historic tragedies.

NATURAL DISASTERS

The federal government defines natural disasters as major events that can include hurricanes, earthquakes, floods, tornadoes, mudslides, snowstorms, or major fires.[3] When a governor determines that a state cannot alone deal with a disaster, the federal government is drawn into the picture. In response to a governor's request for help, the president issues a disaster declaration. Records dating back to 1953 identify more than twenty-six hundred major disaster declarations.[4] The highest number of declarations was in 2011 and included many Appalachian states. Major disaster declarations generally cover large areas with multiple counties, and sometimes entire states, so major disaster declarations are imperfect indicators of their severity in the Appalachian region. Despite this, we can get a sense of the overall impact of disasters in the region by looking at Appalachian areas of states during specific time periods.

Disaster declarations are based on their magnitude combined with the inability of states and local places to manage the situation. It is not surprising that Appalachian states have been subject to a relatively high number of these declarations. Limited resources in regard to emergency response, environmental health, and infrastructure contribute to the likelihood that a single weather event or chemical release will become a major event. Furthermore, major disaster declarations will likely continue as the impacts of climate change emerge throughout Appalachia and include more severe and more frequent extreme weather events such as floods.

Disaster declarations due to flooding are common in Appalachian states, and some of the nation's most tragic and historic floods have occurred in the region. It is easy to find local people who want to talk about the floods they have endured. Flooding is not unique to Appalachia, but several characteristics make the region more prone to floods than other places.[5] First, regional geography lends itself to severe flooding. When communities are in deep valleys between hills, even minor flash flooding can have major impacts. Second, seemingly minor rainfall can create significant environmental health problems because of a lack of capacity for rapid response. Third, industry in the region relies on water for transporting goods, diluting pollution, and storing waste. This increases the potential for exposure to chemicals and pathogens that could seriously affect public health during a flood.

Not surprisingly, many of the most damaging floods result from a combination of natural and human forces. In these hybrid disasters, nature provides the water and people create the circumstances for flood waters to cause environmental health impacts. Dams and impoundments found throughout Appalachia are time bombs that are detonated by the weather. The National Inventory of Dams includes more than thirty thousand dams in the thirteen states of Appalachia and the average age of these dams is fifty-seven.[6] At the very least, environmental destruction is likely when dams fail, but the Army Corps of Engineers classifies about 70 percent of them as either "high" or "significant" hazards, meaning human life is at stake if they fail. Old, shoddily built, and poorly maintained dams are key factors in some of the most devastating floods in Appalachia. This includes the great Johnstown, Pennsylvania, flood of 1889, which is one of the worst flood disasters in the nation's history.

I am connected to historic Johnstown floods because of the time I spent there as a child. My grandmother's house in Johnstown was at the top of a steep hill overlooking a massive railroad switching yard. My sisters, cousins, and I spent a lot of time at a window on the second-floor landing, watching trains. When we would go into town, we could see the high-water marks from the 1889 and 1936 floods. Everyone who lived in Johnstown in the 1960s and 1970s, including my aunts and uncles, told harrowing stories about floods. As an astounding combination of natural and human forces, the 1889 Johnstown Flood remains to this day a formidable symbol of devastating catastrophes in Appalachia.

Johnstown, in western Pennsylvania, was central to steel manufacturing in the late 1800s. The steel industry thrived there because of the town's proximity to natural resources, including iron ore, coal, and wood. The robust demand for steel allowed Johnstown to grow from about five thousand people in 1852 to more than thirty thousand by 1890. Steel brought jobs and jobs brought people. As the city's population exploded, the steel it produced expanded the railroad system across the country and attracted other industries.[7] Like many towns in Appalachia, rivers flow through the valley at Johnstown, and the waterways serve as both transportation routes and pollution catchments. Johnstown's geography contributed to flooding on a regular basis, as riverbanks overflowed during heavy rains. In an uncannily predictive way, one that foreshadows a pattern of environmental inequities throughout the Appalachian region, the historic 1889 flood was caused by a dam built to benefit those who would not be affected by its breach.

Steel barons and other entrepreneurs, many of whom were from Pittsburgh, built the Salt Fork Fishing and Hunting Club in the hills above Johnstown. They designed the club to be a vacation spot for elites who were turning Johnstown into an industrial center. The wealthy out-of-towners wanted a lake to enhance their recreational experience, so they built a dam, without oversight from any regulatory agency. When an engineer tried to warn club patrons that the dam was not safe, they ignored him and kept on using the lake.[8] On May 31, 1889, the dam burst during a heavy rain, flooding Johnstown with millions of gallons of water and killing 2,209 people.[9] Stories of this flood's aftermath detail the human suffering. The stories also highlight community efforts to work together to rescue neighbors, recover the dead, and, eventually, rebuild the town. The 1889 Johnstown Flood represents environmental injustice at its core, a century before we came to understand and document its effects. This flood stands as a prominent example of how socioeconomic status leads one group to harm another group for personal benefit.

Almost one hundred years after the 1889 Johnstown Flood, the circumstances of another historic flood in Logan County, West Virginia, were similar to those in Johnstown. In what is known as the Buffalo Creek disaster, breaches in three dams constructed from coal waste, or gob, caused this catastrophe. When heavy rain inundated the county in late February 1972, the dams failed, unleashing a torrent of water into the nearby communities. More than 132 million gallons of wastewater flooded into the valley without warning. An estimated 125 people died, at least a thousand were injured, and thousands in the towns along Buffalo Creek became homeless in a matter of minutes.

Unlike Johnstown, the dams that burst in the Buffalo Creek flood were not built so that rich people could swim and fish. Their construction was for an industrial rather than a recreational purpose, but the resemblances between these two events are glaring. In both cases, a combination of natural forces and a failure of human-made structures caused the flood. In both cases, the dams did not benefit those who lived in harm's way. In both cases, their construction resulted in disproportionate impacts to vulnerable people, who ultimately suffered the most from the floods.

These historical floods offer a warning of future disasters for many places in Appalachia. As the climate changes, the region is projected to become wetter and warmer. If these projections are proven true, Appalachian people will be among the most vulnerable to the impacts of climate change because of their geography, reliance on the environment, lack of response capacity, and subpar health status. The Intergovernmental Panel on Climate Change (IPCC) notes in its special report on disasters that "exposure and vulnerability are key determinants of disaster risk and of impacts when risk is realized."[10] In many ways, because of social determinants of health, including a legacy of resource depletion, climate change is creating conditions that will heighten the potential for disasters in the region.

Climate Change

The National Research Council, which includes the National Academy of Sciences, the National Academy of Engineering, and the National Academy of Medicine (formerly the Institute of Medicine), summarized the scientific basis for climate change in the 2010 report *Advancing the Science of Climate Change*.[11] The report lays out the indisputable, documented scientific information related to changing climate. Thermometers are not the only indicator that the earth is getting warmer: evidence exists in ecological changes on land, in the oceans, and around glaciers. Humans are causing the climate to change in ways that cannot be explained by natural processes alone, and emissions of gases from burning fossil fuels are the main contributor to the relatively rapid changes.

Climate projections are largely based on observed historical climate indicators such as temperature and precipitation measurements. Such quantitative data are the basis for a variety of models that use scenarios to estimate future climate conditions. Most models use the scenarios, which include a variety of possible levels of future emissions, population growth, and economic conditions, combining sets of these possibilities into distinct projections about the future of the climate for a given region. The scenario selected for a model will affect projections of global and local climate. For example, scenarios that include continued growth in emissions of greenhouse gases result in different projections than a scenario with lower emissions. Despite the wide range of projection possibilities and regardless of the scenario selected, most models suggest that even if dramatic policy measures are taken today, the climate will continue to change into the foreseeable future.

Scientific projections of climate change impacts also suggest regional variability. It is important to look at localized impacts, which can differ significantly from place to place. Some areas will see more precipitation than normal, while others will receive less. Models also show that some regions within countries will get warmer while other areas will cool off. NOAA monitors indicators of climate change in the United States in real time and compiles the data into a cumulative history of change.[12] Their data show that the average annual temperature in most of the United States is increasing. Some years, certain regions in the country have posted lower-than-average temperatures, but, overall, we are in a warming trend.

Regional variations suggest an enhanced environmental and public health burden in Appalachia. Many places in the region are ill equipped to handle major disasters, and the natural effects of climate change will only serve to heighten these events. Even minor variations in average temperatures and precipitation patterns could lead to extensive environmental health effects. According to the United States Geological Survey (USGS), models indicate that the average maximum temperatures in the United States will rise in all states between 2050 and 2074, with a corresponding increase in the average minimum temperature.[13] This means that the United States will generally have warmer days and warmer nights.

Projected changes in the average temperatures in the Appalachian states may not be as great as in the Southwest or upper Midwest, but they are likely to be greater than those experienced in the southern and southeastern states. Increases in average annual temperatures could have some positive effects in some areas in Appalachia, including longer growing seasons. However, warmer average temperatures could also intensify some of the existing public health conditions in the region, including asthma. Overall, the USGS estimates that the average annual changes in precipitation will increase slightly in most of the country, except in the southwest and parts of southern California. The Appalachian states might see modest increases in rain but may also have modest reductions in snow.

The precipitation and temperature projections in Appalachia might seem inconsequential; however, even small changes could lead to more extreme weather events. In place that is already vulnerable, there will be inevitable new challenges to the public health system. The National Climate Assessment shows that the eastern United States has already seen major changes in precipitation since 1958.[14] Environmental health personnel will face challenges ensuring that people in Appalachia are prepared for the consequences of climate change. Public perceptions about climate change continue to perplex scientists who have documented changes and modeled projections. Even though a clear majority of Americans believe the climate is changing, only about half of Americans think climate change is mostly caused by humans.[15] People who live in the Appalachian region tend to be even more skeptical of humans' role in climate change.

In addition, many Americans still think that there is a lot of disagreement among scientists about climate change. In general, Americans are split on how worried they are about climate change, but those in Appalachian states appear to be a little less worried than in some other regions of the country, particularly the west coast and northeast. West Virginians are the most skeptical about climate change, the least worried about it, and not supportive of any strategies that reduce the country's reliance on coal to address climate change.[16] These perceptions create quite a conundrum, because it is likely that West Virginians will be among those most vulnerable to projected climate-change impacts.

Climate Justice

As a noted author, environmental activist, and founder of 350.org, a climate change movement, Bill McKibben refers to climate change as an accidental environmental issue. He sees it more as an example of what happens in an "unequal society."[17] He explains that people who have contributed the least to the problem are already suffering the most. For example, developing countries producing almost no greenhouse gas emissions are currently experiencing climate change that threatens their health and livelihoods. International scientists agree that future disproportionate effects from climate change will become more pronounced and extreme events such as floods and droughts will affect places that are already vulnerable. Climate change is becoming an additional environmental inequity for vulnerable communities. As such, it will become a major contributor to health disparities due to its potential for creating place-based environmental health conditions.

Representatives of some marginalized communities have already started to take notice. The projected disproportionate impacts have led organizations like the National Association for the Advancement of Colored People to focus more keenly on climate justice.[18] Climate justice is related to environmental justice by drawing attention to the disproportionate impacts that befall low-income and minority communities. Climate justice is at the center of an international movement that is raising awareness about inequities already existing between places. Some places will be more affected by climate elements such as weather extremes, disease-spreading insects, and water shortages. With climate change, these inequities will increase, deepen, and widen existing health disparities.

The international movement of front-line communities most vulnerable to the impacts of climate change emerged during a 2014 climate justice summit organized by the Climate Justice Alliance. The summit was held in conjunction with the United Nations Climate Summit and the People's Climate March. This summit included sessions focusing on the current effects of climate change on low-income communities, indigenous populations, and communities of color across the globe. The summit as well as the Climate Justice Alliance is giving a voice to vulnerable people in places that will face the brunt of climate change's impacts on environmental health—at least in urban areas and developing countries.

In spring 2015, environmental health authorities in the US government were paying attention to the climate justice movement. The National Institute of Environmental Health Sciences (NIEHS) hosted a conference on climate justice. Conference discussion revolved around the disproportionate impacts on people in developing countries and communities of color, especially in urban areas in the United States. The plight of low-income rural areas in the United States was largely lacking from the discussion—a troubling indicator of the inability of some public health experts to see environmental inequities in rural places. Appalachia is made up of rural places disproportionately vulnerable to climate change. As their history shows, Appalachian communities are susceptible to weather-related disasters, and the increasing magnitude and frequency of these events will create more environmental and public health problems.

At the 2015 NIEHS conference on climate justice, the organization's director of extramural research and training said that climate change is "not an emerging health threat anymore, it is a real health threat."[19] She went on to note that those who are already subject to disproportionate impacts from environmental conditions will suffer the most as climate change affects local areas. Getting Appalachian communities that are beholden to the fossil fuel–based economy ready for climate change impacts is almost impossible, and sometimes dangerous. There are still people in specific Appalachian places who think climate change is a hoax, even though the science gets more certain every day. In these places people continue to fight for expanding coal mining and reducing regulations for burning it. Paradoxically, it might be these places where climate change will ultimately cause the greatest health impacts.

As politicians and public health officials disregard the potential for catastrophic impacts from climate change in Appalachia, scientists are not helping either. Appalachia's vulnerability to climate change is pushed further into the shadows in how projections are demarcated on a map of the country. In the instances when regional data exists and climate projections are available, the states that comprise Appalachia are delineated as being part of two or more regions. For example, the United States Global Climate Research Program includes Ohio in the Midwest region; New York, Pennsylvania, West Virginia, and Maryland in the Northeast region; and Virginia, Kentucky, Tennessee, Alabama, Mississippi, North Carolina, South Carolina, and Georgia in the Southeast region.[20] These regions are used in the congressionally mandated National Climate Assessment and by government agencies such as the EPA to make projections about environmental impacts of climate change.[21] There are no projections for the Appalachian region nor are there estimates for impacts in rural versus urban areas.

The ecological climate change impacts on Appalachia have been examined more than the health impacts.[22] Assessing potential future influences of changing temperatures and rainfall on plant species and habitat is critical in understanding the overall picture of climate change including its health impacts. There are some species in Appalachia that may suffer from changes in average temperatures and precipitation, while others may benefit. For example, pollen is likely to increase in response to warmer temperatures and longer growing seasons. Scientists generally agree that increases in exposures to pollen are likely to result in an additional public health burden from allergies, asthma, and even chronic obstructive pulmonary disease (COPD).[23] As with many public health impacts, those who are least able to cope with what could be serious respiratory conditions are the most vulnerable to climate change impacts.

Human vulnerability to climate change involves more than just being exposed to its effects. It is a function of exposure, sensitivity, and adaptive capacity. People in many places may be fine if they are healthy and have resources to adapt and respond. A wealthy community with good access to health care and adequate infrastructure will recover much quicker than a poor community without these amenities. Look at the difference between recovery from Hurricane Sandy on the East Coast and Hurricane Maria in Puerto Rico to see how socioeconomic and environmental conditions magnify vulnerability. Multimillion-dollar homes along the Jersey Shore were rebuilt quickly, while people in Puerto Rico waited months to have their power restored. People who live in Appalachia may need to cope with increases in heat-related air pollutants such as pollen and ozone, mosquitoes bringing new diseases to the region, and weather events even more extreme and more disastrous than those in the past. Low-income rural places will struggle due to a lack of resources for adapting to climate change and its short- and long-term effects.[24]

Climate and Environmental Health

Environmental impacts related to climate change have been examined for decades, but human health issues only hit the radar of public health professionals recently. In 2010, the NIEHS summarized research needs for examining the human health impacts of climate change.[25] It specifically addressed the need for research on eleven health conditions: asthma and respiratory allergies; cancer; cardiovascular disease and stroke; foodborne diseases and nutrition; heat-related morbidity and mortality; developmental effects; mental health; neurological diseases and disorders; vector-borne and zoonotic diseases; waterborne diseases; and weather-related morbidity and mortality. Appalachian people already experience some of the highest rates in the country of many of these conditions. The increasing prevalence of asthma, for example, is among the most important public health issues in Appalachia and across the United States.

In 2016, almost 26 million Americans reported that they had been diagnosed at some time with asthma, representing more than 8 percent of the country's population.[26] If you live below the poverty line, you are more likely to have asthma, especially if you are under the age of eighteen. States in the Appalachian region have higher-than-average rates of adult asthma, as well as of asthma-related deaths. Current asthma prevalence makes it a significant public health concern that affects quality of life, leads to premature mortality, and fosters economic and social disruption.

Climate change has the potential to increase the overall burden of asthma across the United States, but especially in Appalachia. There are environmental conditions that trigger acute asthma attacks and otherwise affect those with chronic asthma symptoms. Warming temperatures enhance conditions for certain air pollutants that exacerbate asthma, particularly ground-level ozone. Ozone near the ground is the same chemical compound present in the ozone layer that is protecting us from the harmful cancer-causing solar radiation in the upper atmosphere. When it forms close to the ground, ozone becomes part of smog. Unlike other air pollutants, ozone is not emitted from a specific source; rather, a chemical reaction in the presence of heat and sunlight forms ozone. Without heat as a catalyst for the reaction, ozone levels can remain manageable. Public health alerts and consequences related to ozone increase as temperatures increase.

Smog also includes microscopic particles in the air, or particulate matter (PM). In the thirteen states that comprise Appalachia, those counties within the boundaries of Appalachia have significantly higher levels of particulate matter than those outside the boundaries.[27] Particulate matter is emitted from vehicles and industrial and electricity-generating facilities, especially those burning coal. Coal mining has also been documented as a source of PM because of the dust generated during the process, and this is especially problematic in those places where mountaintop-removal mining is prevalent. Particulate matter is a major health concern because the superfine particles often contain harmful chemicals that can become lodged in the respiratory system, leading to chronic as well as acute health effects.

UNNATURAL DISASTERS

Imagine that an earthquake has caused the top of a mountain to slide off into the valleys and streams below it. Earthquakes scare people, and the government might even get involved to examine the impacts of such a natural disaster on the local environment and health. Now imagine that someone sets an explosive to blast off the top of same mountain, with the same effects. In this case, the government has been complicit in creating a tragic and unnatural disaster. Mountaintop-removal mining (MTR) is an important unnatural, or human-made, disaster. Mountaintop removal only happens in Appalachia, specifically in the central region that includes Kentucky, West Virginia, Virginia, and Tennessee.

MTR is a relatively cheap and easy way to mine coal without sending people underground. Mining companies use explosives to shear off entire mountaintops to reach a seam of coal. The part of the mountain that is destroyed, referred to as overburden, is pushed into valleys and streams below. MTR creates a range of environmental impacts. Some of these are localized, like acid mine drainage. Others are regional, like a warmer climate because the MTR sites will reflect less of the sun's energy back to atmosphere than the forests they replaced, potentially leading to a heat island effect. In addition, forests serve as sinks for carbon compounds, and replacing them with grassland further exacerbates climate change.

MTR operations are required to obtain permits from state regulatory agencies prior to site excavation. Companies must also obtain permits to push overburden into the valleys and streams below. The permitting process is complicated, involving the Army Corps of Engineers (USACE), the EPA, and other federal, state, and local environmental departments. The USACE is the key agency enabling MTR, because it issues permits under the Clean Water Act to manage dredge and fill materials that will be put in waterways. There are several general permits for specific types of activities that do not require more detailed review. The USACE views MTR as one of these activities, thus allowing mining companies to efficiently obtain permits under the nationwide program. This was the case in 1997, when the USACE issued a general permit to a subsidiary of Arch Coal to use two hollows in West Virginia as disposal sites for the largest proposed MTR mining operation in history.

The Spruce No. 1 Surface Mine was designed to spread across more than three thousand acres, and plans were to shove the overburden into Pigeonroost Hollow, a place with some of the highest-quality streams in the state. Almost immediately, people who lived in the hollow began filing lawsuits to stop the project. It was clear that they could not rely on their elected officials to protect them from the pending unnatural disaster. In 1999, a federal district court granted an injunction, saying that the harms to the plaintiffs would be "imminent and irreversible."[28] The judge acknowledged that there would be economic impacts to the coal company, but that these would be short-term and did not outweigh the threats to the people in the area.

In settling one of the lawsuits, the USACE agreed to complete a voluntary Environmental Impact Statement (EIS) to examine impacts of MTR in the coalfields in central Appalachia. The public announcement about the EIS noted that

The number of mountaintop mining operations that utilize valley fills, as well as the scale of individual operations, have increased in recent years in West Virginia. This EIS will evaluate significant environmental impacts associated with these operations on water quality, streams, aquatic and terrestrial habitat, habitat fragmentation, the hydrological balance, and other individual and cumulative effects. Federal and state agencies are increasingly concerned over the lack of comprehensive data regarding valley fill operations, and have initiated a number of studies to address these data gaps. Accurately describing and quantifying the extent and nature of direct, secondary, and cumulative impacts related to valley fills and associated mining practices is difficult.[29]

This sounded promising, in that the federal government appeared ready to identify the environmental impacts of MTR after decades of approving of the practice. Then, George W. Bush was elected president. In 2005, the federal agencies punted on the EIS and issued a Programmatic Environmental Impact Statement (PEIS) on MTR in Appalachia.[30] Instead of evaluating the environmental impacts of the mining, the PEIS looked at how all the agencies involved in regulating MTR worked together. In fact, the PEIS touts the coal resources in central Appalachia and focuses on how to make the permitting process for MTR more efficient for coal companies.

The Army Corps of Engineers issued a new permit to Arch Coal for the project at Spruce No. 1 mine in 2007, using the general permitting provision of the Clean Water Act—the one that did not require the company to apply for an individual permit for the site. Environmental groups immediately filed a lawsuit, but mining got underway in the meantime. President Obama took office in 2009, and in September the EPA sent a letter to the USACE requesting that the permit be invalidated. Under the new administration, the EPA believed there were obvious environmental impacts from MTR and they wanted to study and document what these impacts are. The USACE was not happy with the request and did not intend to comply with it.

In March 2010, the EPA used its veto power under the Clean Water Act for the first time in history. It overruled the USACE, prohibiting use of the valleys below the Spruce No. 1 mine as disposal sites. In January 2011, the EPA made a final determination that there would be no overburden allowed in the streams below the mining site. The people who lived in the hollow breathed a sigh of relief for the first time after almost fifteen years of stress. Politicians in West

Virginia and Washington, DC, were enraged and emboldened by the action and declared this part of Obama's war on coal. Even after a lawsuit and appeals, the January 2011 determination stands, and the Spruce No. 1 mine has not expanded as planned.

Although mountaintop-removal mining is still occurring in central Appalachia, it has declined since 2008.[31] This decline is likely more related to the decreasing market for coal than to resistance by environmentalists or concern about public health. In the meantime, the environmental health impacts of MTR on Appalachia are irreversible and have been compared to volcanic eruptions.[32] In May 2011, the EPA published a report that looked at several hundred studies about MTR in Central Appalachia.[33] The report summarized significant impacts to water and land habitats that include filling (and destroying) wetlands and polluting streams with minerals. While the report focused on examining existing environmental impacts related to MTR, it pointed out that there are environmental effects likely to influence human health as well.

MTR is emerging as a significant source of air pollution in Appalachia. Chemicals in airborne particles are associated with coal geology and these particles are higher in areas with MTR than in areas with subsurface or no mining.[34] This is important because some of these chemicals are linked to asthma and other respiratory conditions. Even with only a few published research studies, the potential for respiratory and cardiovascular health outcomes related to MTR intensifies the health disparities in the region.[35]

MTR is a human-made, unnatural disaster in central Appalachia. The waste it creates changes the topography of the area, making it more prone to flooding. Other ways to manage coal-related waste are also disastrous. One of these techniques is the surface impoundment, or coal-ash pond. These ponds are found throughout Appalachia. The EPA calls these ponds "coal combustion residuals (CCR) surface impoundments" and identifies coal ash as one of the most significant sources of industrial waste in the United States.[36]

Coal combustion residuals include several by-products of burning coal. Fly ash is the lightweight material that would drift out of smokestacks while coal is burned if it wasn't captured through pollution control equipment. Bottom ash is the remains of the coal not completely burned, like the residue left in a charcoal grill after a cookout. There are two ways to deal with coal ash: it is repurposed into construction products such as cement, concrete, and wallboard; or it is managed on site. The only way to deal with fly ash is to use water, because the ash is so light when it is dry that it floats into the air like embers at a campfire.

Despite regulation and monitoring, accidents happen at coal-ash ponds. When these occur, they can be disastrous to the environment and human health.

In the Public Health Assessment of the 2008 Kingston coal-ash spill, the Tennessee Department of Health notes that the timing of the spill probably saved lives.[37] Because it was December, people were not on the river in their boats or outside engaging in recreation activities. The Public Health Assessment summarizes a range of health effects immediately following the spill. At the time of the spill, drinking-water wells in the area did not show unusual levels of the substances found in fly ash, such as heavy metals. The assessment did identify health effects from air pollution, mainly in relation to cleanup activities.

The most significant health effects noted were related to mental health. Many people close to the spill said they were anxious and stressed about it, probably having some of the same fears and worries that people who live below MTR sites do. Most people who were surveyed did not identify any changes in their health other than anxiety, although survey data indicated a relationship between proximity to the site and changes in physical health. Specifically, those who lived closest to the spill were more likely to report coughing, vomiting, and stress than those who lived further away.

We cannot know now whether there will be long-term health effects from the Kingston spill. However, it led the EPA to conduct a countrywide assessment of coal-ash ponds to get a sense of the dangers that these impoundments might pose.[38] The assessment identified more than 640 different units storing, holding, or disposing of coal combustion residuals. The ponds were rated using FEMA's guidelines for dam safety, based on the potential impact of a breach on the surrounding community. Of the 640 ponds, thirty-two were rated as having a high hazard potential, meaning that a breach would probably cause a loss of human life. Of the thirty-two, thirteen are in Appalachian counties.

One of these high-hazard ponds, owned by Duke Energy, is in western North Carolina. This facility was the focus of a lawsuit in which Duke Energy pleaded guilty to violating the Clean Water Act and agreed to pay a $68 million criminal fine and $34 million on projects to improve the local environment.[39] Criminal charges were filed against the company when a major ash spill occurred at one of their facilities in North Carolina. While government investigators sought information about this spill, known as the Dan River Spill, they uncovered a history of environmental crimes at other Duke plants. Duke illegally polluted water sources with coal ash for a long time before the spill exposed their practices.

The largest coal-ash pond in the country straddles the Pennsylvania and West Virginia border. It is the 1,900-acre Little Blue Run pond in Beaver County, Pennsylvania, and Hancock County, West Virginia. The pond was built in 1976–77 and stores coal-ash waste from one power plant in Shippingport, Pennsylvania. This impoundment was also rated high hazard, based on the impacts should the dam fail. There is concern that the Blue Run is leaking and could be contaminating groundwater.[40] Even though the Little Blue Run pond closed in 2012, this enormous coal-ash pond will remain an environmental health problem for years to come.

PLACE OF FUTURE OF DISASTERS

Clearly, there are significant concerns related to the current and future impacts of both natural and unnatural disasters in Appalachia. Environmental health professionals can learn a great deal from the history of floods to help prepare for projected climate change. In addition, officials can use the disasters related to the coal industry to prepare for potential disasters from natural gas exploration. Are any of these historic disasters currently helping public health officials build capacity for a future that may further impair the health of Appalachian people? Probably not. The fight between environmental health and economic development wages on.

In a region already burdened with pollutants exacerbating asthma and other respiratory health effects, climate change will compound and worsen health disparities. In Appalachia, activities in the region, specifically coal mining, are contributing to global changes that will ultimately lead to local human health issues. Shale gas and oil extraction will also likely deepen health disparities. Unfortunately, we are even further behind in examining the public health effects of these processes than we were with MTR. It will be many years before conclusive studies estimate the magnitude of the human health impacts from the rush to extract shale gas in Appalachia. Meanwhile, the current data related to asthma and other respiratory diseases indicate that even small changes in average temperatures and local weather conditions are likely to increase the suffering of people in the region. The potential for health impacts from natural and unnatural disasters remains high in Appalachia.

Epilogue

Ailing in Place

Beautiful, a beautiful [area] that's severely exploited with the remnants
of ruined communities everywhere. You know, whatever energy
companies have come in, created jobs, you know, allowed people to
have enough money to start a family, buy a pick-up truck—and then
left, and people can't afford a dentist or, you know, other basic services
they're after, and they kind of live in poverty and hopelessness. But,
Appalachian people are some of the strongest, hardest workers that
I've ever met, you know. I'm so impressed by them. And yet, there's
this, you know, this other element, you know, that just leaves them in,
you know, dire straits. So it's a very interesting mix.

—Impression of Appalachia from thirty-five-year resident

APPALACHIA IS A PLACE OF PARADOXES. IT HAS SOME OF THE
country's most treasured environmental amenities, but also some of the worst
environmental health. The environment is both naturally beautiful and unnat-
urally dangerous. There are places in Appalachia like none other on earth, with
diverse species, clear water, amazing mountains, fresh air, and exciting options
for outdoor recreation. There are also local places in the region with some of
the highest levels of pollution in the United States and the most unsafe water.
These perplexing contradictions contribute both positively and negatively to
the health of the people who live here.

Overall, Appalachian people are not only less wealthy than those in
many other places in the United States, they are also less healthy. Many of the

well-known health disparities in the region are related to behaviors, such as diet-related diabetes and smoking-related lung disease. However, we cannot explain the health disparities in the region as the result of individual actions alone. Systemic poverty, inadequate education, high rates of unemployment, and abysmal environmental conditions share the blame for the poor health status of people who live in Appalachia. I hope the issues and stories highlighted in this book have brought a new perspective on the range of environmental inequities in Appalachia and how these inequities can affect health. I also hope to highlight the challenges environmental health professionals face in protecting public health in Appalachia. Many of the stories told in this book were identified by those who know the region because they work here, live here, or both.

While researching this book, it became abundantly clear that Appalachia is a place where people are less healthy than other places. It is also a place where it is imperative to understand the impact of the environment on health. Even those exposures found in other places, such as air pollution, have greater health impacts in Appalachia because of underlying social circumstances. Appalachia is a place with distinctive environmental circumstances that disproportionately affect the people who live here. We have documented environmental injustice and inequities in urban areas, and it is time to focus our efforts on doing the same in rural areas. "Evidence-based" is a term that has entered the field of public health. It means that there is data to support policy decisions and prevention programs. In general, there is not enough evidence to fully grasp how environmental conditions contribute to health outcomes, let alone health disparities.

Even with inconsistencies and evidence gaps, there are specific environmental health conditions in Appalachia that reveal health disparities not explained by behaviors alone. These conditions create exposure inequities, especially among people who live in rural places in the region.

- Flooding is prominent in Appalachia. Kentucky and West Virginia rank among the top five states for flood-disaster declarations, even though they are not coastal states like Texas, which ranks number one.

- The largest human-caused or unnatural disasters are tied to places in Appalachia, including the coal-ash spill in Kingston, Tennessee, and the Elk River chemical spill in Charleston, West Virginia.

- Coal mining kills more workers in Appalachia than in all other states combined. Almost 85 percent of the coal mining fatalities since 2004 have taken place in Appalachian mines, mostly in West Virginia.

- Mountaintop-removal mining occurs only in Appalachia. The environmental and health impacts of this practice are irreversible and include mental health effects.

- Appalachian counties consistently rank among the top twenty-five counties for pollution released into the environment from industry. The facilities reporting releases in Appalachia are larger and employ fewer people on average than those outside the region.

- Food security is a serious concern in Appalachia, and most of the states with the highest need of government food assistance are in the region. Food-safety challenges are also of concern due to the number of outbreaks of foodborne illnesses and the lack of adequate resources to manage and prevent them.

- Appalachian states contribute a significant amount to national air pollution emissions, accounting for at least one-third of all the emissions of carbon dioxide, sulfur dioxide, and nitrogen dioxides.

- Two of the three Department of Energy sites used to enrich uranium are in rural Appalachian counties as delineated by the Appalachian Regional Commission. The third is just outside the boundaries of Appalachia but in an Appalachian state.

- Of the coal-ash impoundments identified as high risk by the federal government, about one-third are in Appalachia. In addition, the largest coal-ash impoundment in the country is in Appalachia.

- Appalachian counties are less likely than other places to be covered by statewide smoking bans, a situation contributing to the highest smoking rates in the country.

There are specific inequities in environmental conditions and exposures noted throughout this book. It is probably even more telling that almost all of the Appalachian environmental health professionals I surveyed for background perceive environmental conditions in Appalachia to be worse than in the rest of the country. These are the people who work in Appalachian places, so their knowledge and perceptions of conditions are invaluable. The professionals who participated in the survey as well as those I interviewed are most concerned about private drinking-water systems, private wastewater systems, and the built environment. They also believe that there are health disparities and environmental injustice in Appalachia. They have seen it firsthand.

Many of the unique environmental exposures in Appalachia are related to the coal industry. These include the water impacts from the early coal camps as well as disasters from how coal ash is managed. These historic problems with coal are part of the consequences from the singular emphasis on addressing economic disparities in Appalachia. The economy is the number one consideration in transportation planning, land-use decisions, and permitting and promoting new industries in many local places. It appears that elected officials in the region have tunnel vision and are willing to improve the economy at all cost, including costs related to the environment and health.

Coal is not the only contributor to health disparities in Appalachia, but it gets a lot of attention in research. Researchers trying to explain why people are unhealthy also tend to focus on lifestyle and health behaviors. This book is meant to highlight factors and conditions that are not specifically related to behaviors but are contributing to health disparities. Harmful behaviors do contribute a great deal to the health status of Appalachian people. The evidence indicates that people here smoke more, eat worse, and exercise less than people in other places. With this evidence in hand, public health agencies spend their limited resources on trying to change behaviors. Smoking cessation, nutrition policies, and exercise incentive programs can certainly work to improve public health. However, even if every person in Appalachia changed to a healthier lifestyle, there would still be factors beyond individual behaviors affecting their health.

These nonbehavioral social determinants of health in Appalachia include significant environmental exposures from deliberate past and current activities in the region. There are also exposures resulting from unknown or unintended consequences of decisions and actions. For example, inside places expose people, especially children, to radon, lead, and secondhand smoke. Of these three exposures, behavioral programs are only able to modify smoking. Radon and lead exposures must be eliminated by modifying the built environment. This is a more intense and daunting task than encouraging people to quit smoking. Place-based environmental aspects contribute to health disparities where Appalachian people live, work, and play. These aspects are among the determinants of health that are extremely important to understand and measure.

Even though there are notable environmental differences between Appalachian and non-Appalachian places, inequities in environmental exposures have not been well-documented. At least part of the reason for this is our focus on treatment rather than prevention. We emphasize curing people once they are sick and dismiss opportunities for environmental health interventions. Rural Appalachia takes a one-two punch, because people get knocked down when they are sick and, as they try to get up, lack of access to health care knocks them down again. Local public health departments stand outside of the ring, waiting to be tagged in, but never are. There is not enough money for widespread prevention in a world where the economy runs on a profit-driven health care system.

At the local level, competition between the economy and environmental health continues to affect planning decisions. These decisions focus on ribbon-cutting initiatives, such as building new highways, opening industrial facilities, and drilling new gas wells. The only word that needs to be uttered to justify a new environmental assault is "jobs." The stories in this book do not corroborate the economic benefits that were promised to the places where projects were located. While interviewing in Appalachia, I sensed that people are getting a little weary and wary of these promises. Much of the fatigue is based in worry about documented environmental and health impacts outweighing the undocumented economic ones. Stories of local places and the broader empirical evidence suggest that the overall health of people who live in Appalachia has not benefited from decisions that were meant to bring economic development. Even if there have been short-term economic gains, the long-term health of Appalachians in many places has suffered.

Even without specific studies and data documenting environmental inequities, there are indicators pointing to a wide range of inequitable exposures in Appalachia. The environmental health impacts from the coal industry are the most prominent, apparent in acid mine drainage, poor air quality, and unnatural disasters. Not as prominent are those conditions that stem from an aging water infrastructure, inadequate access to reliable and safe food, deteriorating housing, and a lack of resources for local environmental health activities and programs. In addition, climate change and more extreme weather events will create additional inequitable environmental health impacts in Appalachia.

Unlike environmental health inequities, health disparities have been well documented in Appalachia. What is still missing is a body of research that scientifically validates the link between environmental exposures and health. This research is likely to remain elusive for many reasons. The nature of environmentally related illnesses is such that many of them, for instance cancer, are chronic and linked to myriad factors. However, when a place has the highest rates of a specific type of cancer and the highest amount of reported releases of toxic pollutants, we should examine the connection between the two.

The difficulty in making a connection between environmental exposures and health disparities in Appalachia is also due to the intense power of economic disparities in the region. After decades of work to reduce all disparities, whether regarding health or the economy, there is still much to be done. Many local places are one plant closing away from becoming a community identified as "distressed" by the Appalachian Regional Commission. As informative as it is to label a place in this manner, it does not help mitigate the real impacts on the health of the people who live in these distressed and unhealthy places. This fact sustains my belief that it might not be possible to have both a thriving economy and a clean environment in some rural Appalachian places. Here, decision makers are blinded by any project that might improve the economy, especially if they can attach some estimates of new jobs created. Until economic conditions improve for whatever reason, the health of many rural Appalachians remains in jeopardy.

Despite decades of gathering and reporting data related to pollution emissions and environmental quality, the accuracy of this data is still evolving. In some cases, there are significant data limitations because of the protocols for reporting releases. In other cases, environmental monitoring is only done when there is a problem or accident. What we are left with is a shortage of data related to background exposures. This is especially problematic when new projects and activities are introduced into an already contaminated environment. If there is no data to show contaminant levels before the project starts, it is impossible to link environmental conditions caused by the activities to health problems.

It is fitting to let Appalachian environmental health professionals have the final word. To complete this discussion of environmental inequities and health disparities in the region, below are some verbatim observations of these professionals as captured in a 2014 survey.

- The intersecting inequalities in Appalachia require public health efforts to consider factors that have not always been included in previous efforts. New technology and new ways of thinking are required; however, there is a large gap in accountability of private industry and the impacts to public health in these regions, particularly in natural resource extraction. Manufacturing and agriculture also have significant impacts in local Appalachian communities, both good and bad.

- Part of my position involves inspecting school cafeterias, and while I believe more food choice diversity is offered, high fructose corn syrup is still in many of the products. Our budget has all but cut the health educator positions and doubled our workload, so we do not have the time to educate—it's all about getting 100 percent of the inspections complete even though we are overlooking the most important component, which is education. I know from attending regional and statewide meetings that the poorer the area, the less EHS [environmental health science] positions are in place—there is no doubt that the health in these areas must suffer as a result of insufficient staff.

- Our state has very different topography in the Appalachian area as compared to the rest of the state. In our state, this area is also very economically depressed and the industry is mostly coal related. The economic climate and the tough terrain and air quality issues associated with their chief economic industry make health issues in this area much worse.

- County health departments in Appalachia have perpetually suffered from a lack of resources and populations there are often underserved. Recent in-migration has improved economic resources some, but the area tends to lag behind the more populous areas of North Carolina.

- Appalachian communities seem to have a limited voice in state government and natural resources are not managed to benefit the local communities.

- The state that I work within has poor management skills and has cut environmental programs. There has been a statewide reduction in workforce on all budgets in the state. When viewing websites from the state, many positions are vacant and not to be filled. The local-level county agencies have cut budgets, which in turn affects budgets of the local health departments. In the smaller-population counties, the local health departments are on the verge of collapse because of funding. I predict that regional health departments will occur in the next five years.

- Appalachia is still the prime area for coal mining and other environment-damaging industries. The residents are primarily poor and rural and not well-educated. Many families are dependent on the father for sustenance, as the mother usually stays home to take care of children. The father might be employed in a dangerous job that might impact his overall health. Many times, the father becomes disabled, further adversely impacting the income of the family. While there are services available to the poor in Appalachia, the rural nature of the area and the remoteness of local communities make it difficult for these services to be delivered, especially in times of emergency. These are people in the greatest need of health care, yet the rural nature of the area makes it hard to sustain a physician in a remote community. Plus, transportation services are not provided to cover rural areas and many poor residents do not own vehicles to travel to doctors and hospitals in larger cities well over an hour away. Thus, many Appalachia residents are in serious jeopardy from what are usually routine health problems in urban areas.

Appendix 1

*Summary of the Environmental Health
Profession in Appalachian States*

State	State environmental health board	Credential required	Professional state association	EH professional title
Alabama	NO	NO	YES	Public Health Environmentalist
Georgia	YES	NO	YES	Registered Environmental Health Professional
Kentucky	YES	YES	YES	Registered Sanitarian
Maryland	YES	YES	YES	Environmental Health Specialist
Mississippi	NO	NO	YES	Public Health Environmentalist
New York	NO	NO	YES	Public Health Sanitarian
North Carolina	YES	YES	YES	Environmental Specialist
Ohio	YES	YES	YES	Registered Sanitarian/ Environmental Health Specialist
Pennsylvania	NO	NO	YES	Sanitarian
South Carolina	YES	NO	YES	Sanitarian
Tennessee	NO	NO	YES	Environmental Health Specialist
Virginia	NO	NO	YES	Environmental Health Specialist
West Virginia	YES	NO	YES	Environmental Inspector

Appendix 2

Summary of State Agency Involvement in
Select Environmental Health Programs

State	State agency	Built environment	Water and wastewater	Food	Pollution	Natural resource extraction	Disasters and climate change
Alabama	Alabama Public Health	X	X	X	X		
	Department of Environmental Management		X		X		
Georgia	Department of Public Health	X	X	X			
	Department of Natural Resources	X	X		X	X	X
Kentucky	Department for Public Health	X	X	X			
	Department for Environmental Protection		X	X			
	Department for Natural Resources					X	
Maryland	Department of Health	X	X	X			
	Department of the Environment	X	X		X	X	X
	Department of Natural Resources		X				
Mississippi	Department of Health	X	X	X			
	Department of Environmental Quality		X		X	X	
New York	Department of Health	X	X	X			X
	Department of Environmental Conservation		X		X	X	X

State	State agency	Built environ-ment	Water and waste-water	Food	Pollution	Natural resource extraction	Disasters and climate change
N. Carolina	Department of Health and Human Services	X	X	X			
	Department of Environmental Quality		X		X	X	X
Ohio	Department of Health	X	X	X			
	Environmental Protection Agency		X		X		X
	Department of Natural Resources		X		X	X	
Pennsylvania	Department of Health	X		X		X	
	Department of Environmental Protection		X		X	X	X
	Department of Conservation and Natural Resources					X	
S. Carolina	Department of Health and Environmental Control	X	X	X	X		
	Department of Natural Resources		X				X
Tennessee	Department of Health	X		X			
	Department of Environment and Conservation		X		X	X	X
Virginia	Department of Health	X	X	X			
	Department of Environmental Quality		X		X	X	X
W. Virginia	Department of Health and Human Resources	X		X			
	Department of Environmental Protection		X		X	X	X

Discussion Questions

1. In thinking about the concept of "place," do you think where you live contributes either positively or negatively to your overall health?

2. There is a difference between inequities and disparities. Discuss this difference.

3. Explain the relationship between poverty, health, and the environment.

4. Is creating a map that shows a relationship between hazardous waste sites and race enough to argue that there is environmental injustice? How would one design a research study to further explore cause and effect rather than just relationships?

5. Warren County, North Carolina, is not in Appalachia. Nevertheless, it was an important place in regard to environmental justice for the region. Why?

6. How has neighborhood design contributed to some of the most prevalent health effects in the United States?

CHAPTER 1: FOUNDATIONS OF ENVIRONMENTAL HEALTH

1. Describe the profession of environmental health.

2. How did cholera contribute to the formation of environmental health? How is cholera an example of a health disparity?

3. Do international public health organizations such as the World Health Organization (WHO) play any role in local public health programs?

4. Based on the information provided in this chapter, why do you think that more attention is paid to global health disparities than to local health disparities?

5. Explain how environmental health is the first line of defense against disease.

6. Discuss the relationship between the US government and local environmental health practice.

7. Did you have any knowledge of the profession of environmental health before reading this chapter? How has your understanding of the field changed after reading it?

8. How does Appalachia manage environmental health programs? Use the case of Ohio's regulatory approach to environmental health to discuss the challenges to managing environmental health at the state and local levels.

9. Why do you think there are resource constraints that make it difficult to fully implement many environmental health programs?

CHAPTER 2: A PLACE FOR THE BUILT ENVIRONMENT AND HEALTH

1. Throughout the book, a common theme emerges about decisions made to reduce economic disparities in Appalachia. How have these decisions contributed to health disparities in the region?

2. The County Health Rankings are noted in this chapter. Go to the website that houses these rankings (https://www.countyhealthrankings.org) and look up the county that is your home. Are you surprised by some of the information that is found there?

3. Discuss the relationship between planning and public health. Which came first? How has this relationship evolved through history?

4. What do you think has contributed to the emphasis on addressing public health issues in urban areas rather than rural areas in the United States?

5. Explain why radon is such an important environmental health issue.

6. How is exposure to lead different from exposures to other heavy metals such as arsenic and mercury? How are these exposures similar?

7. How does the smoking rate in Appalachia contribute to health disparities among children in the region? Why is it challenging to address the public health impacts of smoking in Appalachia?

8. Transportation planning is identified in this chapter as creating both positive and negative health effects in Appalachia. Identify one of each type of effect.

CHAPTER 3: A PLACE FOR WATER

1. Discuss how the legacy of coal mining has affected drinking water in some communities in Appalachia.

2. What factors contribute to widespread public attention to major water-contamination episodes in Appalachia, while a large percentage of people there have no or limited regular access to any clean water?

3. Has the emphasis on improving public drinking-water and wastewater systems in Appalachia made a difference in improving private water management?

4. What impact has the situation with federal funding of water improvements had on water quality in Appalachia?

5. Explain the challenges in maintaining water quality from surface water sources versus groundwater sources.

6. Do you think that there will be long-term public health consequences from the Elk River spill? Why or why not?

7. How might the Elk River spill improve the safety of water quality in the entire country?

8. Which do you think is more important, addressing drinking-water or wastewater infrastructure?

9. Why is it a significant challenge to manage private wastewater treatment systems?

CHAPTER 4: A PLACE FOR FOOD

1. Discuss the role of farmers' markets in addressing food security in Appalachia.

2. What is the food paradox in Appalachia? Is there a solution to this paradox?

3. What challenges do farmers' markets create for environmental health professionals responsible for ensuring food safety?

4. What is the relationship between food security and obesity? Discuss how this relationship affects people in Appalachia.

5. How can food-related health outcomes such as diabetes and obesity contribute to a lack of food safety in Appalachia?

6. Locate one foodborne outbreak in an Appalachian county and discuss how local environmental health professionals responded to the outbreak.

7. Why is changing requirements for the national school lunch program so controversial?

8. How has the local-foods movement contributed to food safety issues in retail establishments such as restaurants?

CHAPTER 5: A PLACE FOR POLLUTION

1. What made small communities in Appalachia attractive to the federal government as it sought locations for uranium enrichment?

2. How did the 1979 accident at Three Mile Island affect the Portsmouth Gaseous Diffusion Plant (PORTS) in Pike County, Ohio?

3. Discuss the role that the government plays in facility-siting decisions. Use the case of municipal landfills as an example.

4. Do you think that Appalachia meets the criteria to be considered a pollution haven in the United States?

5. What is your opinion about the role that local zoning ordinances might have on the location of hazardous facilities?

6. How has the discourse related to jobs and environment contributed to the pollution-haven hypothesis?

7. How would you design a research project to prove that exposure to pollution causes negative health effects?

8. Is there enough evidence to indicate that pollution has contributed to health disparities in Appalachia?

CHAPTER 6: A PLACE FOR RESOURCE EXTRACTION

1. What are some of the factors that have contributed to the decline of coal as a major component of the economy in Appalachia? Do you think there is any one factor that has played the most significant role?

2. How did the federal government become involved in mine safety?

3. Younger miners in Appalachia are beginning to show signs of black lung disease. What impact might this have on the future of mining?

4. Did the federal government play a role in the Upper Big Branch mining disaster? Why are some mines with multiple safety violations allowed to stay open?

5. Discuss the public health impacts from the lifecycle of coal.

6. How are the cases of Imboden, Virginia, and Cheshire, Ohio, similar? How are they different?

7. What role do economic conditions play in hydraulic fracturing activity?

8. Since research related to public health impacts from hydraulic fracturing is "slim," should local governments continue to encourage this process in their communities? What alternatives do they have?

9. Why do you think the EPA halted monitoring activities in Pavillion, Wyoming?

10. Compare and contrast the environmental, health, and economic issues related to coal versus natural gas.

CHAPTER 7: A PLACE FOR DISASTERS

1. Explain how the 1972 Buffalo Creek flood in West Virginia was similar to the 1889 flood in Johnstown, Pennsylvania.

2. Why is Appalachia vulnerable to climate change?

3. Do you agree with the distinction the author makes between natural and unnatural disasters? Are all disasters natural? Why even make this distinction?

4. How has the coal industry contributed to disasters in Appalachia?

5. What is climate justice? How does Appalachia fit into the discussion of climate justice?

6. Bill McKibben says climate change is an "accidental" environmental issue. What does this mean?

7. Discuss the impact of asthma in Appalachia, including the current and future public health burdens from this disease.

8. The Public Health Assessment for Kingston, Tennessee, was completed in 2010 and noted very few health impacts from the spill. What are your thoughts about these findings, considering the magnitude of the disaster?

9. Coal-ash ponds are a major way to manage ash at coal-fired power plants. Should they be? If not, how should this waste be managed?

10. In your opinion, what is the most important type of future disaster that Appalachian people should prepare for now?

Notes

INTRODUCTION TO APPALACHIAN PLACE AND HEALTH

1. United Health Foundation, *America's Health Rankings: 2018 Annual Report* (Minnetonka, MN: United Health Foundation, 2018), https://www.americashealthrankings.org/learn/reports/2018-annual-report.

2. "Social Determinants of Health," Office of Disease Prevention and Health Promotion, US Department of Health and Human Services, last modified July 3, 2019, https://www.healthypeople.gov/2020/topicsobjectives2020/overview.aspx?topicid=39.

3. Paula Braveman and Susan Egerter, *Overcoming Obstacles to Health in 2013 and Beyond* (Princeton, NJ: Robert Wood Johnson Foundation, 2013), https://www.rwjf.org/en/library/research/2013/06/overcoming-obstacles-to-health-in-2013-and-beyond.html.

4. Regarding geography, see James Howard Kunstler, *The Geography of Nowhere: The Rise and Decline of America's Man-Made Landscape* (New York: Touchstone, 1993). Regarding identity, see Tracy Kidder, *Home Town* (New York: Pocket Books, 2000). Regarding childhood, see Richard Louv, *Last Child in the Woods: Saving Our Children from Nature-Deficit Disorder* (Chapel Hill, NC: Algonquin, 2008).

5. Rudy Abramson and Jean Haskell, "Introduction," in *Encyclopedia of Appalachia*, ed. Abramson and Haskell (Knoxville: University of Tennessee Press, 2006), xxi.

6. Phillip J. Obermiller, "Thoughts on the Importance of Identifying Appalachians," *Appalachian Journal* 38, no. 1 (2010): 62–64.

7. Appalachian Regional Development Act of 1965, Pub. L. No. 89-4, 40 U.S.C. § 141 (1965).

8. Ann DeWitt Watts, "Does the Appalachian Regional Commission Really Represent a Region?," *Southeastern Geographer* 18, no. 1 (1978): 19–36.

9. Secretary's Advisory Committee on National Health Promotion and Disease Prevention Objectives for 2020, *Phase I Report: Recommendations for the Framework and Format of Healthy People 2020* (Washington, DC: Department of Health and Human Services, 2008), https://www.healthypeople.gov/sites/default/files/PhaseI_0.pdf.

10. Centers for Disease Control and Prevention, "CDC Health Disparities and Inequalities Report—United States, 2011," *Morbidity and Mortality Weekly Report* 60, supplement (January 14, 2011): 1–116, https://www.cdc.gov/mmwr/pdf/other/su6001.pdf.

11. Centers for Disease Control and Prevention, "CDC Health Disparities and Inequalities Report—United States, 2013," *Morbidity and Mortality Weekly Report* 62, no. 3, supplement (November 22, 2013): 1–186, https://www.cdc.gov/mmwr/pdf/other/su6203.pdf.

12. Michigan Civil Rights Commission, *The Flint Water Crisis: Systemic Racism through the Lens of Flint* (Detroit: Michigan Department of Civil Rights, 2017), 55, https://www.michigan.gov/documents/mdcr/VFlintCrisisRep-F-Edited3-13-17_554317_7.pdf.

13. "Poor Physical Health Days," America's Health Rankings, accessed June 13, 2017, https://www.americashealthrankings.org/explore/2016-annual-report/measure/PhysicalHealth/state/ALL.

14. "Behavioral Risk Factor Surveillance System," Centers for Disease Control and Prevention, accessed June 13, 2017, https://www.cdc.gov/brfss/index.html.

15. PDA, Inc. and Cecil G. Sheps Center for Health Services Research, *Health Care Costs and Access Disparities in Appalachia* (Washington, DC: Appalachian Regional Commission, 2012), https://www.arc.gov/assets/research_reports/HealthCareCostsandAccessDisparitiesinAppalachia.pdf.

16. Appalachian Regional Commission, *Investing in Appalachia's Future: The Appalachian Regional Commission's Five-Year Strategic Plan for Capitalizing on Appalachia's Opportunities* (Washington, DC: Appalachian Regional Commission, 2015), https://www.arc.gov/images/newsroom/publications/sp/InvestinginAppalachiasFutureARCs2016-2020StrategicPlan.pdf.

17. Community and Economic Development Initiative of Kentucky, *Program Evaluation of the Appalachian Regional Commission's Health Projects, 2004–2010* (Washington, DC: Appalachian Regional Commission, 2015), https://www.arc.gov/assets/research_reports/ProgramEvaluationofARCsHealthProjects2004-2010.pdf.

18. Julie L. Marshall et al., *Health Disparities in Appalachia* (Washington, DC: Appalachian Regional Commission, 2017), https://www.arc.gov/assets/research_reports/Health_Disparities_in_Appalachia_August_2017.pdf.

19. "Measles Cases and Outbreaks," Centers for Disease Control and Prevention, accessed June 14, 2017, https://www.cdc.gov/measles/cases-outbreaks.html.

20. Paula Braveman, "What Are Health Disparities and Health Equity? We Need to Be Clear," *Public Health Reports* 129, supp. 2 (January–February 2014): 5–8.

21. David Blackley, Bruce Behringer, and Shimin Zheng, "Cancer Mortality Rates in Appalachia: Descriptive Epidemiology and an Approach to Explaining Differences in Outcomes," *Journal of Community Health* 37, no. 4 (August 2012): 804–13, https://doi.org/10.1007/s10900-011-9514-z; Lawrence Barker, Richard Crespo, Robert B. Gerzoff, Sharon Denham, Molly Shrewsberry, and Darrlyn Cornelius-Averhart, "Residence in a Distressed County in Appalachia as a Risk Factor for Diabetes, Behavioral Risk Factor Surveillance System, 2006–2007," *Preventing Chronic Disease* 7, no. 5 (September 2010): 1–9, https://www.cdc.gov/pcd/issues/2010/sep/09_0203.htm.

22. "Current Cigarette Smoking among Adults in the United States," Centers for Disease Control and Prevention, accessed April 7, 2016, https://www.cdc.gov/tobacco/data_statistics/fact_sheets/adult_data/cig_smoking.

23. Keith J. Zullig and Michael Hendryx, "Health-Related Quality of Life among Central Appalachian Residents in Mountaintop Mining Communities," *American Journal of Public Health* 101, no. 5 (May 2011): 848–53.

24. Commission for Racial Justice, *Toxic Wastes and Race in the United States* (New York: United Church of Christ, 1987).

25. "Toxic Wastes and Race at Twenty, 1987–2007," United Church of Christ, March 2007, accessed September 4, 2015, https://www.ucc.org/environmental-ministries _toxic-waste-20.

26. Executive Order 12898 of February 11, 1994, "Federal Actions to Address Environmental Justice in Minority Populations and Low-Income Populations," accessed April 7, 2016, https://www.archives.gov/federal-register/executive-orders/pdf /12898.pdf.

27. Institute of Medicine, Committee for the Study of the Future of Public Health, *The Future of Public Health* (Washington, DC: National Academies Press, 1988), 40.

28. "Ten Great Public Health Achievements in the 20th Century," Centers for Disease Control and Prevention, accessed February 22, 2015, https://www.cdc.gov/about /history/tengpha.htm.

29. "Overweight and Obesity," Centers for Disease Control and Prevention, accessed February 22, 2015, https://www.cdc.gov/Obesity.

CHAPTER 1: FOUNDATIONS OF ENVIRONMENTAL HEALTH

1. World Health Organization, *The First Ten Years of the World Health Organization: 1948–1957* (Geneva: World Health Organization, 1958), https://www.who.int /global_health_histories/who_history/en/.

2. Hugh S. Cumming, "The International Sanitary Conference," *American Journal of Public Health* 16, no. 10 (October 1926): 975–80; Norman Howard-Jones, *The Scientific Background of the International Sanitary Conferences 1851–1938*, History of International Public Health 1 (Geneva: World Health Organization, 1975), https://apps.who.int/iris /handle/10665/62873.

3. John Snow, *Snow on Cholera: Being a Reprint of Two Papers* (New York: Commonwealth Fund, 1936), 18, https://pds.lib.harvard.edu/pds/view/7291561.

4. Steven Johnson, *The Ghost Map: The Story of London's Most Terrifying Epidemic— and How It Changed Science, Cities, and the Modern World* (New York: Riverhead Books, 2007).

5. "Constitution," World Health Organization, accessed July 29, 2019, https:// www.who.int/about/who-we-are/constitution.

6. "World Health Assembly Endorses the Rio Political Declaration on Social Determinants of Health," World Health Organization, June 26, 2012, https://www.who.int /sdhconference/background/en/.

7. World Health Organization and UNICEF, *Progress on Drinking Water and Sanitation: 2014 Update* (Geneva: World Health Organization, 2014), 6, https://www.who.int /water_sanitation_health/publications/2014/jmp-report/en/.

8. E. Corcoran, C. Nellemann, E. Baker, R. Bos, D. Osborn, H. Savelli, eds., *Sick Water? The Central Role of Wastewater Management in Sustainable Development* (Arendal, Norway: UNEP/UN-HABITAT/GRID-Arendal, 2010), https://www.grida.no/publications/218.

9. "Household Air Pollution and Health," World Health Organization, last modified May 8, 2018, https://www.who.int/mediacentre/factsheets/fs292/en/.

10. Pan American Health Organization, *The Pan American Sanitary Code: Toward a Hemispheric Health Policy* (Washington, DC: Pan American Health Organization, 1999), 1, http://www1.paho.org/hq/dmdocuments/2008/code-1999.pdf.

11. Pan American Health Organization, *Strategic Plan of the Pan American Health Organization 2014–2019: Championing Health: Sustainable Development and Equity* (Washington, DC: Pan American Health Organization, 2014), 106, http://iris.paho.org/xmlui/handle/123456789/7654.

12. United Nations Development Programme and United Nations Environment Programme, "Joint Programme Proposal: Joint UNDP-UNEP Poverty-Environment Initiative 2013–2017," June 2013, 1, https://www.unpei.org/sites/default/files/dmdocuments/PEI_PRODOC_2013-2017.pdf.

13. Institute of Medicine, Committee on Public Health Strategies to Improve Health, *For the Public's Health: Investing in a Healthier Future* (Washington, DC: National Academies Press, 2012), https://iom.nationalacademies.org/Reports/2012/For-the-Publics-Health-Investing-in-a-Healthier-Future.aspx.

14. "Key Features of the Affordable Care Act by Year," National Center for Biotechnology Information, accessed July 30, 2019, https://www.ncbi.nlm.nih.gov/books/NBK241401/.

15. Institute of Medicine, Committee on Public Health Strategies to Improve Health, *For the Public's Health*.

16. National Institute of Environmental Health Sciences, *2018–2023 Strategic Plan: Advancing Environmental Health Sciences, Improving Health*, NIH Publication No. 18-ES-7935 (Bethesda, MD: National Institutes of Health, 2018), 2, https://www.niehs.nih.gov/about/strategicplan/index.cfm.

17. National Institute of Environmental Health Sciences, 7.

18. "Food Safety—High Risk Issue," US Government Accountability Office, accessed July 30, 2019, https://www.gao.gov/key_issues/food_safety/issue_summary.

19. See appendix 2.

20. Robert Jay Dilger, *Unfunded Mandates Reform Act: History, Impact, and Issues*, CRS Report R40957 (Washington, DC: Congressional Research Service, 2015), last updated August 28, 2019, https://www.fas.org/sgp/crs/misc/R40957.pdf.

21. Personal interviews with state environmental health professionals; websites and resources provided by state organizations and agencies (see appendix 1).

22. Matt McKillop and Vinu Ilakkuvan, *The Impact of Chronic Underfunding of America's Public Health System: Trends, Risks, and Recommendations, 2019* (Washington, DC: Trust for America's Health, 2019), https://www.tfah.org/report-details/2019-funding-report/.

CHAPTER 2: A PLACE FOR THE BUILT ENVIRONMENT AND HEALTH

1. "Pennsylvania Department of Corrections Monthly Population Report as of October 30, 2019," https://www.cor.pa.gov/About Us/Statistics/Documents/current monthly population.pdf.

2. "SCI Forest," Pennsylvania Department of Corrections, accessed September 26, 2015, https://www.cor.pa.gov/Facilities/StatePrisons/Pages/Forest.aspx.

3. "Pennsylvania: Forest (FO)," County Health Rankings & Roadmaps, Robert Wood Johnson Foundation, accessed August 1, 2019, https://www.countyhealthrankings.org/app/pennsylvania/2019/rankings/forest/county/outcomes/overall/snapshot.

4. Forest County Community and Economic Development Department, "2016 Three Year Community Development Plan (CDP)," 6, http://www.co.forest.pa.us/departments/docs/CDP 2016 Final.docx.

5. "Pennsylvania Prison Construction 2011–2014," Decarcerate PA, accessed September 26, 2015, https://decarceratepa.info/sites/default/files/PA_Prison_Expansion_Map_2011-2014.pdf.

6. "2015–16 Fiscal Year Cost Per Inmate—General Fund," Pennsylvania Department of Corrections, accessed August 13, 2017, https://www.cor.pa.gov/Documents/15-16_cost_per_day.pdf.

7. "QuickFacts: Forest County, Pennsylvania," US Census Bureau, accessed August 1, 2019, https://www.census.gov/quickfacts/forestcountypennsylvania.

8. Forest County Community and Economic Development Department, "2016 Three Year Community Development Plan (CDP)," 6.

9. Forest County Conservation District and Planning Commission Board, *Forest County Comprehensive Plan* (Tionesta, PA: Forest County Commissioners, 2013), 19, http://www.co.forest.pa.us/departments/docs/2013 Forest County Comprehensive Plan.pdf.

10. Forest County Conservation District and Planning Commission Board, 16.

11. Johanna Lemon, "The Great Stink," Cholera and the Thames, accessed August 4, 2019, https://www.choleraandthethames.co.uk/cholera-in-london/the-great-stink/.

12. Jon A. Peterson, "The Impact of Sanitary Reform upon American Urban Planning, 1840–1890," *Journal of Social History* 13, no. 3 (Autumn 1979): 83–103.

13. "Healthy Communities," American Public Health Association, accessed February 22, 2015, https://www.apha.org/topics-and-issues/healthy-communities.

14. "Designing and Building Healthy Places," Centers for Disease Control and Prevention, accessed February 22, 2015, https://www.cdc.gov/healthyplaces/.

15. "Healthy People 2020: Environmental Health," Office of Disease Prevention and Health Promotion, US Department of Health and Human Services, accessed April 11, 2016, https://www.healthypeople.gov/2020/topics-objectives/topic/environmental-health/objectives.

16. Appalachian Regional Commission, "Status of the Appalachian Development Highway System as of September 30, 2016," https://www.arc.gov/images/programs/transp/ADHSStatusReportFY2016.pdf.

17. "Health Impact Assessment," Centers for Disease Control and Prevention, last updated September 19, 2016, https://www.cdc.gov/healthyplaces/hia.htm.

18. "The Health Impact Project," The Pew Charitable Trust, accessed November 28, 2019, https://www.pewtrusts.org/en/projects/health-impact-project/health-impact -assessment.

19. "Indoor Air Quality and Environmental Justice," Environmental Protection Agency, accessed August 4, 2019, https://www.epa.gov/indoor-air-quality-iaq/introduction -indoor-air-quality#justice.

20. Hajo Zeeb and Ferid Shannoun, eds., *WHO Handbook on Indoor Radon: A Public Health Perspective* (Geneva: World Health Organization, 2009), https://www.who.int /ionizing_radiation/env/radon/en/index1.html.

21. Environmental Protection Agency, *The National Radon Action Plan: A Strategy for Saving Lives*, EPA 402/R-15/001 (Washington, DC: Environmental Protection Agency, 2015), https://www.epa.gov/sites/production/files/2015-11/documents/nrap _guide_2015_final.pdf.

22. David Blackley, Bruce Behringer, and Shimin Zheng, "Cancer Mortality Rates in Appalachia: Descriptive Epidemiology and an Approach to Explaining Differences in Outcomes," *Journal of Community Health* 37, no. 4 (August 2012): 804–13, https://doi .org/10.1007/s10900-011-9514-z.

23. "Health Risk of Radon," Environmental Protection Agency, accessed August 4, 2019, https://www.epa.gov/radon/health-risk-radon.

24. Michael Hendryx, Kathryn O'Donnell, and Kimberly Horn, "Lung Cancer Mortality Is Elevated in Coal-Mining Areas of Appalachia," *Lung Cancer* 62, no. 1 (October 2008): 1–7, https://doi.org/10.1016/j.lungcan.2008.02.004.

25. Lene H. S. Veiga, Eliana C. S. Amaral, Didier Colin, and Sérgio Koifman, "A Retrospective Mortality Study of Workers Exposed to Radon in a Brazilian Underground Coal Mine," *Radiation and Environmental Biophysics* 45, no. 2 (July 2006): 125–34, https:// doi.org/10.1007/s00411-006-0046-3.

26. "EPA Map of Radon Zones," Environmental Protection Agency, accessed August 4, 2019, https://www.epa.gov/radon/epa-map-radon-zones.

27. Mountains of Hope Cancer Coalition, *WV Cancer Plan 2016–2020* (Charleston, WV: West Virginia Department of Health and Human Resources, 2016), https://dhhr .wv.gov/hpcd/FocusAreas/wvcancer/Documents/WV_CANCER_PLAN_2016-2020 _FINAL.pdf.

28. Centers for Disease Control and Prevention, "Blood Lead Levels in Children Aged 1–5 Years—United States, 1999–2010," *Morbidity and Mortality Weekly Report* 62, no. 13 (April 5, 2013): 245–48, https://www.cdc.gov/mmwr/preview/mmwrhtml /mm6213a3.htm.

29. "CDC National Childhood Blood Lead Surveillance Data," Centers for Disease Control and Prevention, last update July 30, 2019, https://www.cdc.gov/nceh/lead /data/national.htm.

30. Childhood Lead Poisoning Prevention Program, *2017 Childhood Lead Surveillance Report* (Harrisburg, PA: Pennsylvania Department of Health, 2018), https://www

.health.pa.gov/topics/Documents/Environmental Health/2017 Childhood Lead Surveillance Annual Report.pdf.

31. R. Constance Wiener and Richard J. Jurevic, "Association of Blood Lead Levels in Children 0–72 Months with Living in Mid-Appalachia: A Semi-Ecologic Study," *Rural and Remote Health* 16, no. 2 (April 2106): 1–8, https://www.rrh.org.au/journal/article/3597.

32. "Rural Urban Definitions," Center for Rural Pennsylvania, accessed August 6, 2019, https://www.rural.palegislature.us/demographics_rural_urban.html.

33. Kimberly Yolton, Marie Cornelius, Asher Ornoy, James McGough, Susan Makris, and Susan Schantz, "Exposure to Neurotoxicants and the Development of Attention Deficit Hyperactivity Disorder and Its Related Behaviors in Childhood," *Neurotoxicology and Teratology* 44 (July–August 2014): 30–45, https://doi.org/10.1016/j.ntt.2014.05.003.

34. "Age-Adjusted Invasive Cancer Incidence Rates in Kentucky: All Sites, 2012–2016," Kentucky Cancer Registry, accessed August 6, 2019, https://www.cancer-rates.info/ky/.

35. "United States Cancer Statistics," Centers for Disease Control and Prevention, last updated June 28, 2019, https://www.cdc.gov/cancer/uscs/index.htm.

36. "Economic Trends in Tobacco," Centers for Disease Control and Prevention, last updated July 23, 2019, https://www.cdc.gov/tobacco/data_statistics/fact_sheets/economics/econ_facts/.

37. "Census of Agriculture: 2017 Census by State," United States Department of Agriculture, accessed August 6, 2019, https://www.nass.usda.gov/Publications/AgCensus/2017/Full_Report/Census_by_State/index.php.

38. "Health Effects of Secondhand Smoke," Centers for Disease Control and Prevention, last updated January 17, 2018, https://www.cdc.gov/tobacco/data_statistics/fact_sheets/secondhand_smoke/health_effects/index.htm.

39. Samrat Yeramaneni, Kimberly Yolton, Kurunthachalam Kannan, Kim N. Dietrich, and Erin N. Haynes, "Serum Cotinine versus Parent Reported Measures of Secondhand Smoke Exposure in Rural Appalachian Children," *Journal of Appalachian Health* 1, no. 1 (2019): 15–26, https://www.ncbi.nlm.nih.gov/pmc/articles/PMC6553863/.

40. Amy K. Ferketich, Alex Liber, Michael Pennell, Darren Nealy, Jana Hammer, and Micah Berman, "Clean Indoor Air Ordinance Coverage in the Appalachian Region of the United States," *American Journal of Public Health* 100, no. 7 (July 2010): 1313–18, https://doi.org/10.2105/AJPH.2009.179242.

41. "Map of Smokefree Indoor Air—Private Worksites, Restaurants, and Bars," Centers for Disease Control and Prevention, last updated June 30, 2019, https://www.cdc.gov/statesystem/smokefreeindoorair.html.

42. "Health Disparities Related to Smoking in Appalachia," Appalachian Regional Commission, April 2019, https://www.arc.gov/research/researchreportdetails.asp?REPORT_ID=158.

43. "Diabetes," America's Health Rankings, 2018 Annual Report, accessed November 28, 2019, https://www.americashealthrankings.org/explore/annual/measure/Diabetes.

44. "Health Disparities Related to Obesity in Appalachia," Appalachian Regional Commission, April 2019, https://www.arc.gov/research/researchreportdetails.asp?REPORT_ID=155.

CHAPTER 3: A PLACE FOR WATER

1. Ed Robinson, *Wyoming County*, Images of America Series (Charleston, SC: Arcadia, 2005).

2. "Our Community," Wyoming County Economic Development Authority, accessed August 6, 2019, https://www.wyomingcounty.com/our-community.aspx.

3. "Geography Program," United States Census Bureau, last updated May 16, 2018, https://www.census.gov/geo/reference/gtc/gtc_place.html.

4. Letter from J. D. Douglas, Manager, Compliance and Enforcement Unit, Office of Environmental Health Services, to WV Property LLC, January 11, 2013, accessed August 6, 2019, http://www.psc.state.wv.us/scripts/WebDocket/ViewDocument.cfm?CaseActivityID=379619&NotType='WebDocket'.

5. Jessica Lilly, "After Months Without, Wyoming County Community Gets Safe Water," WV Public Broadcasting, April 23, 2014, https://wvpublic.org/post/after-months-without-wyoming-county-community-gets-safe-water.

6. Carl Hoffman, "A Tale of Two Water Systems," *Appalachia Magazine* 31, no. 1 (January–April 1998): 32–35, available at https://www.arc.gov/magazine/articles.asp?ARTICLE_ID=135&F_ISSUE_ID=17.

7. West Virginia Office of Miners' Health Safety and Training, *2017 Statistical Report and Directory of Mines* (Charleston: West Virginia Department of Commerce, 2017), https://minesafety.wv.gov/PDFs/CY 2017 Annual Report.pdf.

8. "Production of Coal and Coke in West Virginia," West Virginia Office of Miners' Health, Safety, and Training, accessed August 6, 2019, https://minesafety.wv.gov/historicprod.htm.

9. "West Virginia," Bureau of Labor Statistics, accessed August 6, 2019, https://www.bls.gov/regions/mid-atlantic/west_virginia.htm#tab-1.

10. "County-Level Data Sets: Unemployment," United States Department of Agriculture, Economic Research Service, last updated May 30, 2019, https://www.ers.usda.gov/data-products/county-level-data-sets/unemployment.aspx.

11. "QuickFacts: Wyoming County, West Virginia; West Virginia," United States Census Bureau, accessed August 6, 2019, https://www.census.gov/quickfacts/fact/table/wyomingcountywestvirginia,WV/IPE120216#viewtop.

12. "County Data Release 7/23/2019," WorkForce West Virginia, http://lmi.workforcewv.org/DataRelease/CountyRelease.html.

13. "West Virginia: Wyoming (WY)," County Health Rankings & Roadmaps, Robert Wood Johnson Foundation, accessed August 6, 2019, https://www.countyhealthrankings.org/app/west-virginia/2019/rankings/wyoming/county/factors/overall/snapshot.

14. Mark C. Scott, in *Encyclopedia of Appalachia*, ed. Rudy Abramson and Jean Haskell (Knoxville: University of Tennessee Press, 2006), 143–45.

15. "Digitized Mine Maps," Mine Safety and Health Administration, accessed August 16, 2015, https://www.msha.gov/minemapping/minemapping.asp.

16. U.S. Census, "2017 American Housing Survey Data," https://www.census.gov/newsroom/press-releases/2018/ahs.html, accessed November 28, 2019.

17. Government Accountability Office, "Rural Water Infrastructure: Federal Agencies Provide Funding but Could Increase Coordination to Help Communities," statement of Alfredo Gomez, director, Natural Resources and Environment Team, GAO-15-450T, February 27, 2015, https://www.gao.gov/assets/670/668743.pdf.

18. Jeff Hughes, Richard Whisnant, Lynn Weller, Shadi Eskaf, Matthew Richardson, Scott Morrissey, and Ben Altz-Stamm, *Drinking Water and Wastewater Infrastructure in Appalachia: An Analysis of Capital Funding and Funding Gaps* (Chapel Hill: University of North Carolina Environmental Finance Center, 2005), 1–2.

19. The Safe Drinking Water Information System can be accessed at https://www.epa.gov/enviro/facts/sdwis/search.html.

20. "Groundwater Quality in Principal Aquifers of the Nation, 1991–2010," United States Geological Survey, accessed August 6, 2019, https://water.usgs.gov/nawqa/studies/praq/.

21. Evan Hansen, Marc Glass, Ben Gilmer, and Angie Rosser, *The Freedom Industries Spill: Lessons Learned and Needed Reforms* (Morgantown, WV: Downstream Strategies, 2014), https://www.downstreamstrategies.com/documents/reports_publication/freedom-spill-report_1-20-14.pdf.

22. Office of the West Virginia Attorney General, *Elk River Chemical Spill: Incident Report* (Charleston: Office of the West Virginia Attorney General, 2015), https://ago.wv.gov/Documents/010815-ElkRiverChemicalSpill.pdf.

23. Beth Vorhees, "No Concern about Long-Term Health Effects from 2014 Chemical Spill," West Virginia Public Broadcasting, June 16, 2015, https://wvpublic.org/post/no-concern-about-long-term-health-effects-2014-chemical-spill.

24. "All Bill Information (Except Text) for H.R. 2576," United States Congress, accessed August 6, 2019, https://www.congress.gov/bill/114th-congress/house-bill/2576/all-info.

25. Eric Lipton, "Why Has the E.P.A. Shifted on Toxic Chemicals? An Industry Insider Helps Call the Shots," *New York Times*, October 21, 2017, https://www.nytimes.com/2017/10/21/us/trump-epa-chemicals-regulations.html.

26. Office of Wastewater Management, *Primer for Municipal Wastewater Treatment Systems* (Washington, DC: Environmental Protection Agency, 2004), 9, https://www.epa.gov/sites/production/files/2015-09/documents/primer.pdf.

27. "Clean Watersheds Needs Survey," Environmental Protection Agency, last updated April 1, 2019, https://www.epa.gov/cwns.

28. South Carolina did not provide data for the report.

29. Downstream Strategies, *An Assessment of Natural Assets in the Appalachian Region: Water Resources* (Washington, DC: Appalachian Regional Commission, 2014), https://www.arc.gov/assets/research_reports/AssessmentofNaturalAssetsintheAppalachian Region-WaterResources.pdf.

30. Hughes et al., *Drinking Water and Wastewater Infrastructure in Appalachia*.

31. "Wyoming County," Coal Heritage, accessed August 6, 2019, https://coalheritage .org/DocumentCenter.aspx?id=71.

32. West Virginia University Land Use and Sustainable Development Law Clinic, *Wyoming County Comprehensive Plan* (Pineville, WV: Wyoming County Economic Development Authority, 2017), accessible via https://www.wyomingcounty.com/planning -commission.aspx.

CHAPTER 4: A PLACE FOR FOOD

1. Ohio Development Services Agency Research Office, *The Ohio Poverty Report, February 2019* (Columbus: Ohio Development Services Agency, 2019), https://www .development.ohio.gov/files/research/p7005.pdf.

2. "30 Mile Meal," Athens County Visitors Bureau, accessed August 6, 2019, https:// athensohio.com/category/30-mile-meal/.

3. "Ohio: Food Environment Index," County Health Rankings & Roadmaps, Robert Wood Johnson Foundation, accessed August 6, 2019, https://www.countyhealthrankings .org/app/ohio/2019/measure/factors/133/map.

4. "Food Environment Atlas: Go to the Atlas," United States Department of Agriculture, Economic Research Service, last modified July 24, 2019, https://www.ers.usda .gov/data-products/food-environment-atlas/go-to-the-atlas.aspx.

5. James R. Veteto, Gary Paul Nabhan, Regina Fitzsimmons, Kanin Routson, and DeJa Walker, eds., *Place-Based Foods of Appalachia: From Rarity to Community Restoration and Market Recovery* (N.p.: Renewing America's Food Traditions Alliance, 2011), https:// garynabhan.com/pbf-pdf/AA_APPALACHIA'S_PLACE-BASED_FOODS.pdf.

6. "Food Security in the U.S.," United States Department of Agriculture, Economic Research Service, last modified September 5, 2018, https://www.ers.usda.gov/topics /food-nutrition-assistance/food-security-in-the-us/.

7. "Definitions of Food Security," United States Department of Agriculture, Economic Research Service, last modified September 5, 2018, https://www.ers.usda.gov /topics/food-nutrition-assistance/food-security-in-the-us/definitions-of-food-security .aspx.

8. "Food Environment Atlas," United States Department of Agriculture, Economic Research Service.

9. Kirsten A. Grimm, Latetia V. Moore, and Kelly S. Scanlon, "Access to Healthier Food Retailers—United States, 2011," *Morbidity and Mortality Weekly Report* 62, no. 3, supplement (November 22, 2013): 20–26, https://www.cdc.gov/mmwr/preview /mmwrhtml/su6203a4.htm.

10. "Food Insecurity in Ohio," Feeding America, accessed August 7, 2019, https:// map.feedingamerica.org/county/2017/overall/ohio.

11. Feeding America, *Map the Meal Gap 2017: Highlights of Findings for Overall and Child Food Insecurity* (Chicago: Feeding America, 2017), https://www.feedingamerica .org/research/map-the-meal-gap/2015/2015-mapthemealgap-exec-summary.pdf.

12. Karen Cunnyngham, *Reaching Those in Need: Estimates of State Supplemental Nutrition Assistance Program Participation Rates in 2014* (Alexandria, VA: United States Department of Agriculture, Food and Nutrition Service, 2017), https://fns-prod.azureedge.net/sites/default/files/ops/Reaching2014.pdf.

13. Alana Rhone, Michele Ver Ploeg, Ryan Williams, and Vince Breneman, *Understanding Low-Income and Low-Access Census Tracts across the Nation: Subnational and Subpopulation Estimates of Access to Healthy Food*, Economic Information Bulletin 209 (Washington, DC: United States Department of Agriculture, Economic Research Service, 2019), https://www.ers.usda.gov/publications/pub-details/?pubid=93140.

14. Elizabeth Condon, Susan Drilea, Keri Jowers, Carolyn Lichtenstein, James Mabli, Emily Madden, and Katherine Niland, *Diet Quality of Americans by SNAP Participation Status: Data from the National Health and Nutrition Examination Survey, 2007–2010* (Alexandria, VA: United States Department of Agriculture, Food and Nutrition Service, 2015), https://fns-prod.azureedge.net/sites/default/files/ops/NHANES-SNAP07-10.pdf.

15. "Obesity," America's Health Rankings, accessed August 7, 2019, https://www.americashealthrankings.org/explore/annual/measure/Obesity.

16. Feeding America, *Map the Meal Gap 2017*.

17. Jasbir Kaur, Molly M. Lamb, and Cynthia L. Ogden, "The Association between Food Insecurity and Obesity in Children—The National Health and Nutrition Examination Survey," *Journal of the Academy of Nutrition and Dietetics* 115, no. 5 (May 2015): 751–58, https://dx.doi.org/10.1016/j.jand.2015.01.003.

18. Cheryl D. Fryar, Margaret D. Carroll, and Cynthia L. Ogden, "Prevalence of Overweight and Obesity among Children and Adolescents: United States, 1963–1965 through 2011–2012," September 2014, National Center for Health Statistics, https://www.cdc.gov/nchs/data/hestat/obesity_child_11_12/obesity_child_11_12.pdf.

19. "Adolescent Obesity Prevalence: Trends over Time (2003–2017)," Centers for Disease Control and Prevention, accessed August 7, 2019, https://www.cdc.gov/healthyschools/obesity/obesity-youth.htm.

20. Katelynn E. Weber, Andrea F. R. Fischl, Pamela J. Murray, and Baqiyyah N. Conway, "Effect of BMI on Cardiovascular and Metabolic Syndrome Risk Factors in an Appalachian Pediatric Population," *Diabetes, Metabolic Syndrome and Obesity: Targets and Therapy* 7 (2014): 445–53, https://dx.doi.org/10.2147/DMSO.S68283.

21. "Farmers Markets and Direct-to-Consumer Marketing," United States Department of Agriculture, accessed August 7, 2019, https://www.ams.usda.gov/services/local-regional/farmers-markets-and-direct-consumer-marketing.

22. Vicki A. McCracken, Jeremy L. Sage, and Rayna A. Sage, "Do Farmer's Markets Ameliorate Food Deserts?," *Focus* 29, no. 1 (Spring/Summer 2012): 21–26, https://www.irp.wisc.edu/publications/focus/pdfs/foc291f.pdf.

23. Vicki A. McCracken, Jeremy L. Sage, and Rayna A. Sage, "Bridging the Gap: Do Farmer's Markets Help Alleviate Impacts of Food Deserts?," IRP Discussion Paper no. 1401-12, University of Wisconsin–Madison, Institute for Research on Poverty, April 2012, https://www.irp.wisc.edu/publications/dps/pdfs/dp140112.pdf.

24. "Local Food Directories: National Farmers Market Directory," United States Department of Agriculture, last updated August 6, 2019, https://www.ams.usda.gov /local-food-directories/farmersmarkets.

25. Stephanie B. Jilcott Pitts, Alison Gustafson, Qiang Wu, Mariel Leah Mayo, Rachel K. Ward, Jared T. McGuirt, Ann P. Rafferty, Mandee F. Lancaster, Kelly R. Evenson, Thomas C. Keyserling, and Alice S. Ammerman, "Farmers' Market Use Is Associated with Fruit and Vegetable Consumption in Diverse Southern Rural Communities," *Nutrition Journal* 13, no. 1 (2014): 1–22, https://dx.doi.org/10.1186/1475 -2891-13-1.

26. Jilcott Pitts et al., "Farmers' Market Use Is Associated."

27. Sean C. Lucan, Andrew R. Maroko, Omar Sanon, Rafael Frias, and Clyde B. Schechter, "Urban Farmers' Markets: Accessibility, Offerings, and Produce Variety, Quality, and Price Compared to Nearby Stores," *Appetite* 90 (July 2015): 23–30, https:// dx.doi.org/10.1016/j.appet.2015.02.034.

28. Jeffrey Levi, Laura M. Segal, Robyn Gougelet, and Rebecca St. Laurent, *Investing in America's Health: A State-by-State Look at Public Health Funding and Key Health Facts* (Washington, DC: Trust for America's Health, 2015), https://www.tfah.org/report -details/investing-in-americas-health-a-state-by-state-look-at-public-health-funding-key -health-facts-1/.

29. "Estimates of Foodborne Illness in the United States," Centers for Disease Control and Prevention, last updated November 5, 2018, https://www.cdc.gov /foodborneburden/.

30. "National Outbreak Reporting System (NORS)," Centers for Disease Control and Prevention, last updated December 7, 2018, https://www.cdc.gov/nors/.

31. "Help Prevent the Spread of Highly Contagious 'Stomach Bug' (Norovirus)— May 2013," National Park Service, accessed September 16, 2015, https://www.nps.gov /appa/learn/news/index.htm.

32. "Four Multistate Outbreaks of Human *Salmonella* Infections Linked to Live Poultry in Backyard Flocks (Final Update)," Centers for Disease Control and Prevention, last updated July 31, 2015, https://www.cdc.gov/salmonella/live-poultry-07-15 /index.html.

33. Gordon W. Gunderson, *The National School Lunch Program: Background and Development* (Washington, DC: US Government Printing Office, 1971), https://fns-prod .azureedge.net/sites/default/files/NSLP-Program%20History.pdf.

34. Child Nutrition Programs—Income Eligibility Guidelines, 80 Fed. Reg. 17026 (March 31, 2015).

35. Table 204.10 in "Digest of Education Statistics," National Center for Education Statistics, accessed August 7, 2019, https://nces.ed.gov/programs/digest/d15/tables /dt15_204.10.asp.

36. Elizabeth Condon, Susan Drilea, Carolyn Lichtenstein, James Mabli, Emily Madden, and Katherine Niland, *Diet Quality of American School Children by National School Lunch Program Participation Status: Data from the National Health and Nutrition Examination Survey, 2005–2010* (Alexandria, VA: United States Department of Agriculture,

Food and Nutrition Service, 2015), https://www.fns.usda.gov/sites/default/files/ops/NHANES-NSLP05-10.pdf.

37. Nutrition Standards in the National School Lunch and School Breakfast Programs, 77 Fed. Reg. 4083 (January 26, 2012).

38. ICF Incorporated, "Proposed Rule on Meal Pattern Requirements and Nutrition Standards in the National School Lunch Program and School Breakfast Program, Final Summary of Public Comments," October 13, 2011, https://www.regulations.gov/#!documentDetail;D=FNS-2007-0038-64675.

39. "2019 Position Paper," School Nutrition Association, accessed August 7, 2019, https://schoolnutrition.org/legislation-policy/action-center/2019-position-paper/.

40. Marion Nestle, "The School Nutrition Association's Bizarre Saga Continues," *Food Politics* (blog), February 17, 2015, https://www.foodpolitics.com/2015/02/the-school-nutrition-associations-bizarre-saga-continues; Karen Perry Stillerman, "The School Nutrition Association—Opposing Better Nutrition in Schools Since 2013," *The Equation* (blog), Union of Concerned Scientists, April 1, 2015, https://blog.ucsusa.org/the-school-nutrition-association-opposing-better-nutrition-in-schools-since-2013-689.

41. "National Outbreak Reporting System (NORS)," Centers for Disease Control and Prevention, last updated December 7, 2018, https://wwwn.cdc.gov/norsdashboard/.

42. Laura M. Segal and Alejandra Martín, *A Funding Crisis for Public Health and Safety: State-by-State Public Health Funding and Key Health Facts, 2017* (Washington, DC: Trust for America's Health, 2017), https://www.tfah.org/report-details/a-funding-crisis-for-public-health-and-safety-state-by-state-public-health-funding-and-key-health-facts-2017/.

CHAPTER 5: A PLACE FOR POLLUTION

1. "Local Impact of the Plant," Portsmouth Gaseous Diffusion Plant Virtual Museum, accessed August 7, 2019, http://www.portsvirtualmuseum.org/impact3.htm.

2. Kenneth M. McCaffree, "Collective Bargaining in Atomic-Energy Construction," *Journal of Political Economy* 65, no. 4 (August 1957): 322–37.

3. "Nuclear Explained: U.S. Nuclear Industry," US Energy Information Administration, last reviewed April 19, 2019, https://www.eia.gov/energyexplained/index.cfm?page=nuclear_use.

4. Bryan L. Williams, Sylvia Brown, and Michael Greenberg, "Determinants of Trust Perceptions among Residents Surrounding the Savannah River Nuclear Weapons Site," *Environment & Behavior* 31, no. 3 (May 1999): 354–71, https://doi.org/10.1177/00139169921972146.

5. Amy Sheridan, "National Security Exemptions in Federal Pollution Laws," *William & Mary Environmental Law and Policy Review* 19, no. 2 (1995): 287–315, https://scholarship.law.wm.edu/wmelpr/vol19/iss2/5/.

6. State of Ohio v. US Department of Energy, Joint Request for Entry of Consent Decree, US District Court, Southern District of Ohio, Eastern Division, August 29, 1989.

7. Chuck Johnston and Susan Scutti, "Ohio Town Worries about Safety after Radioactive Contamination Is Found at Middle School," May 14, 2019, CNN Health, https://www.cnn.com/2019/05/14/health/ohio-middle-school-radioactivity-bn/index.html.

8. "Ohio: Pike (PK)," County Health Rankings & Roadmaps, Robert Wood Johnson Foundation, accessed August 7, 2019, https://www.countyhealthrankings.org/app/ohio/2019/rankings/pike/county/outcomes/overall/snapshot.

9. 40 C.F.R. 26, Part 258 (2011–12), accessed August 7, 2019, https://www.gpo.gov/fdsys/pkg/CFR-2012-title40-vol26/xml/CFR-2012-title40-vol26-part258.xml#seqnum258.10.

10. Raymond MacDermott, "A Panel Study of the Pollution-Haven Hypothesis," *Global Economy Journal* 9, no. 1 (2009): 1–12, https://dx.doi.org/10.2202/1524-5861.1372.

11. Todd L. Matthews, "The Enduring Conflict of 'Jobs versus the Environment': Local Pollution Havens as an Integrative Empirical Measure of Economy versus Environment," *Sociological Spectrum* 31, no. 1 (2010): 59–85, https://doi.org/10.1080/02732173.2011.525696.

12. Matthews, "The Enduring Conflict of 'Jobs versus the Environment.'"

13. Michele Morrone and Tania B. Basta, "Public Opinion, Local Pollution Havens, and Environmental Justice: A Case Study of a Community Visioning Project in Appalachian Ohio," *Community Development* 44, no. 3 (2013): 350–63, https://doi.org/10.1080/15575330.2013.797005.

14. David M. Konisky and Tyler S. Schario, "Examining Environmental Justice in Facility-Level Regulatory Enforcement," *Social Science Quarterly* 91, no. 3 (September 2010): 835–55.

15. Village of Euclid, Ohio v. Ambler Realty Co., 272 U.S. 365 (1926).

16. Euclid v. Ambler, 390.

17. Peter Roff, "The War on Coal Is Just the Beginning," *US News & World Report*, August 12, 2015, https://www.usnews.com/opinion/blogs/peter-roff/2015/08/12/the-war-on-coal-and-the-clean-power-plan-are-just-the-beginning.

18. See chapter 6 for a more complete discussion of fracking.

19. "2016 TRI National Analysis: Where You Live," Environmental Protection Agency, accessed August 7, 2019, https://gispub.epa.gov/trina2016/.

20. Michele Morrone, Natalie A. Kruse, and Amy E. Chadwick, "Environmental and Health Disparities in Appalachian Ohio: Perceptions and Realities," *Journal of Health Disparities Research and Practice* 7, no. 5 (2014): 67–81, https://digitalscholarship.unlv.edu/jhdrp/vol7/iss5/5.

21. "TRI Basic Data Files: Calendar Years 1987–2017," Environmental Protection Agency, accessed August 7, 2019, https://www.epa.gov/toxics-release-inventory-tri-program/tri-basic-data-files-calendar-years-1987-2017.

22. Daniel Moore, "DEP, Shell Share Air Quality Plans for Beaver County Cracker Plant," *Pittsburgh Post-Gazette*, May 5, 2015, https://powersource.post-gazette.com/powersource/companies/2015/05/05/Public-meeting-addresses-Royal-Dutch-Shell-chemical-plant-proposal-in-Monaca/stories/201505050212.

23. "Shell Buys Former Zinc Smelter Site for $13.5 Million," WFMJ.com, last updated September 7, 2015, https://www.wfmj.com/story/29335054/shell-buys-former-zinc-smelter-site-for-135-million.

24. "'This Is Going to Be a Game-Changer': Anticipation Building for Proposed Cracker Plant in Beaver County," *Observer-Reporter* (Washington, PA), August 8, 2015, https://www.observer-reporter.com/article/20150808/NEWS01/150809526.

25. "More Workers Needed for Cracker Plant, Unions Gear Up Training," *Marcellus Drilling News* (blog), April 9, 2018, https://marcellusdrilling.com/2018/04/more-workers-needed-for-shell-cracker-plant-unions-gear-up-training/.

26. "Growing U.S. HGL Production Spurs Petrochemical Industry Investment," Energy Information Administration, January 29, 2015, https://www.eia.gov/todayinenergy/detail.cfm?id=19771#tabs_SpotPriceSlider-1.

27. Julie L. Marshall et al., *Health Disparities in Appalachia* (Washington, DC: Appalachian Regional Commission, 2017), https://www.arc.gov/assets/research_reports/Health_Disparities_in_Appalachia_August_2017.pdf.

28. David Blackley, Bruce Behringer, and Shimin Zheng, "Cancer Mortality Rates in Appalachia: Descriptive Epidemiology and an Approach to Explaining Differences in Outcomes," *Journal of Community Health* 37, no. 4 (August 2012): 804–13, https://doi.org/10.1007/s10900-011-9514-z.

CHAPTER 6: A PLACE FOR RESOURCE EXTRACTION

1. Ronald D. Eller, *Uneven Ground: Appalachia since 1945* (Lexington: University Press of Kentucky, 2008), 9.

2. "Clean Up Season," *Big Stone Gap Post*, April 21, 1915, quoting Virginia State Board of Health.

3. Allen Newman, "Department of Environmental Quality: Straight Pipe Issues, Southwest VA" (PowerPoint presentation, May 2010), https://cpcri.net/wp-content/uploads/2014/06/StraightPipeIssues.pdf.

4. Interview with Virginia environmental health manager, June 2, 2014.

5. Presentation provided by Virginia environmental health manager, June 2, 2014.

6. Patrick C. McGinley, "From Pick and Shovel to Mountaintop Removal: Environmental Injustice in the Appalachian Coalfields," *Environmental Law* 34, no. 1 (Winter 2004): 21–106, https://www.jstor.org/stable/43266998.

7. "Trading Point: Central Appalachian (CAPP) Is the Nation's Benchmark Price for Eastern Coal," Energy Information Administration, September 19, 2012, https://www.eia.gov/todayinenergy/detail.cfm?id=8030#.

8. Energy Information Administration, *Annual Coal Report 2018* (Washington, DC: Department of Energy, 2019), https://www.eia.gov/coal/annual/pdf/acr.pdf.

9. "Costs of Transporting Coal to Power Plants Rose Almost 50% in a Decade," Energy Information Administration, November 19, 2012, https://www.eia.gov/todayinenergy/detail.cfm?id=8830; "EIA Projects That U.S. Coal Demand Will Remain Flat for Several

Decades," Energy Information Administration, March 30, 2018, https://www.eia.gov
/todayinenergy/detail.php?id=35572.

10. Gregory Clark and David Jacks, "Coal and the Industrial Revolution, 1700–1869,"
European Review of Economic History 11, no. 1 (April 2007): 39–72. https://doi.org/10.1017
/S1361491606001870.

11. Lowering Miner's Exposure to Respirable Coal Mine Dust, Including Continu-
ous Personal Dust Monitors, 79 Fed. Reg. 24813 (May 1, 2014).

12. David J. Blackley, Cara N. Haldinn, and A. Scott Laney, "Resurgence of Debil-
itating and Entirely Preventable Respiratory Disease among Working Coal Miners,"
American Journal of Respiratory and Critical Care Medicine 190, no. 6 (2014): 708–9, https://
doi.org/10.1164/rccm.201407-1286LE.

13. Douglas E. Pollock, J. Drew Potts, and Gerald J. Joy, "Investigation into Dust
Exposures and Mining Practices in Mines in the Southern Appalachian Region," *Mining
Engineering* 62, no. 2 (2010): 44–49.

14. Centers for Disease Control, "Pneumoconiosis and Advanced Occupational
Lung Disease among Surface Miners—16 States, 2010–2011," *Morbidity and Mortality
Weekly Report* 61, no. 23 (June 15, 2012): 431–34, https://www.cdc.gov/mmwr/preview
/mmwrhtml/mm6123a2.htm?s_cid=mm6123a2_w.

15. Mine Safety and Health Administration, "Mine Disaster Investigations since
2000," accessed August 7, 2019, https://www.msha.gov/data-reports/mine-disaster
-investigations-2000.

16. Mine Safety and Health Administration, "Mine Disaster Investigations since 2000."

17. Mine Safety and Health Administration, "Coal Mining Fatalities by State by
Calendar Year," last updated August 8, 2018, accessed September 2, 2018, https://www
.msha.gov/stats/charts/coalbystates.pdf.

18. Michael Hendryx, Leah Wolfe, Juhua Luo, and Bo Webb, "Self-Reported Cancer
Rates in Two Rural Areas of West Virginia with and without Mountaintop Coal Mining," *Journal of Community Health* 37, no. 2 (April 2012): 320–27, https://doi.org/10.1007
/s10900-011-9448-5; Keith J. Zullig and Michael Hendryx, "Health-Related Quality of
Life among Central Appalachian Residents in Mountaintop Mining Counties," *American Journal of Public Health* 101, no. 5 (May 2011): 848–53, https://dx.doi.org/10.2105
/AJPH.2010.300073.

19. "Rail Traffic Data," Association of American Railroads, accessed August 7, 2019,
https://www.aar.org/data-center/rail-traffic-data.

20. "Green Book: Sulfur Dioxide (2010) Nonattainment Areas by State/County
/Area," Environmental Protection Agency, last updated July 31, 2019, https://www3
.epa.gov/airquality/greenbook/tncty.html.

21. "TRI Explorer: Release Reports," Environmental Protection Agency, last updated April 2019, https://iaspub.epa.gov/triexplorer/tri_release.chemical.

22. Committee on Ground Water Recharge in Surface-Mined Areas, Water Science
and Technology Board, National Research Council, *Surface Coal Mining Effects on Ground
Water Recharge* (Washington, DC: National Academies Press, 1990), 148, https://www
.nap.edu/initiative/committee-on-ground-water-recharge-in-surface-mined-areas.

23. David A. Waples, *The Natural Gas Industry in Appalachia: A History from the First Discovery to the Tapping of the Marcellus Shale*, 2nd ed. (Jefferson, NC: McFarland, 2012), 6.

24. Energy Information Administration, "Drilling Sideways: A Review of Horizontal Well Technology and Its Domestic Application," DOE/EIA-TR-0565, April 1993, https://www.yumpu.com/en/document/view/6011625/drilling-sideways-a-review-of-horizontal-well-technology-eia.

25. Justin McCarthy, "Economy Continues to Rank as Top U.S. Problem," Gallup.com, May 16, 2016, accessed August 7, 2019, https://www.gallup.com/poll/191513/economy-continues-rank-top-problem.aspx?g_source=economy&g_medium=search&g_campaign=tiles.

26. Dominic C. DiGiulio, Richard T. Wilkin, Carlyle Miller, and Gregory Oberley, *Draft: Investigation of Ground Water Contamination near Pavillion, Wyoming* (Ada, OK: Environmental Protection Agency, Office of Research and Development), EPA 600/R-00/000, December 2011, https://www.epa.gov/sites/production/files/documents/EPA_ReportOnPavillion_Dec-8-2011.pdf.

27. "Region 8: Pavillion," Environmental Protection Agency, accessed August 7, 2019, https://www.epa.gov/region8/pavillion.

28. Government Accountability Office, "Oil and Gas: Information on Shale Resources, Development, and Environmental and Public Health Risks," 59, GAO-12-732, published September 5, 2012, https://www.gao.gov/products/GAO-12-732.

29. Tanya Tillet, "Summit Discusses Public Health Implications of Fracking," *Environmental Health Perspectives* 121, no. 1 (January 2013): A15, https://ehp.niehs.nih.gov/121-a15/.

30. Research Triangle Environmental Health Collaborative, *Shale Gas Extraction in North Carolina: Public Health Implications* (Raleigh, NC: Research Triangle Environmental Health Collaborative, 2013), https://environmentalhealthcollaborative.org/wp-content/uploads/2018/02/2012SummitWorkProduct.pdf.

31. Mark A. Latham, "The BP Deepwater Horizon: A Cautionary Tale for CCS, Hydrofracking, Geoengineering, and Other Emerging Technologies with Environmental and Human Health Risks," *William and Mary Law Review* 36, no. 1 (2011): 39.

32. Environmental Protection Agency, *Hydraulic Fracturing for Oil and Gas: Impacts from the Hydraulic Fracturing Water Cycle on Drinking Water Resources in the United States (Final Report)*, EPA/600/R-16/236F (Washington, DC: Environmental Protection Agency, 2016), ES-46, https://cfpub.epa.gov/ncea/hfstudy/recordisplay.cfm?deid=332990.

33. "Business Cycle Dating Committee, National Bureau of Economic Research," National Bureau of Economic Research, July 17, 2003, https://www.nber.org/cycles/july2003.html.

34. "Business Cycle Dating Committee, National Bureau of Economic Research," National Bureau of Economic Research, September 20, 2010, https://www.nber.org/cycles/sept2010.html.

35. "Natural Gas: Number of Producing Gas Wells," Energy Information Administration, last updated July 31, 2019, https://www.eia.gov/dnav/ng/ng_prod_wells_s1_a.htm.

36. "Ohio Oil & Gas Well Locator," Ohio Department of Natural Resources, accessed August 8, 2019, https://oilandgas.ohiodnr.gov/well-information/oil-gas-well-locator.

37. Amanda Woodrum, *Fracking in Carroll County, Ohio: An Impact Assessment* (Cleveland, OH: Policy Matters Ohio, 2014), 3, https://www.policymattersohio.org/wp-content/uploads/2014/04/Shale_Apr2014.pdf.

38. Personal interview, Carroll County Chamber of Commerce representative, June 2013.

39. Woodrum, *Fracking in Carroll County*, 23.

40. Ohio Oil and Gas Energy Education Program, "Estimated Economic Impact from the Utica Shale Geological Formation Only," n.d., https://oogeep.org/wp-content/uploads/2013/02/Economic-Impact-Study-Estimated-Utica-Shale-2011-Final.pdf.

41. Scott Suttell, "Reuters Says Shale's Impact on Job Creation in Ohio Is Disappointing," blog post, June 14, 2013, Crain's Cleveland Business, accessed September 20, 2015, https://www.crainscleveland.com/article/20130614/BLOGS03/130619840/-1/blogs03.

42. Amanda Woodrum, "Executive Summary," April 10, 2014, Policy Matters Ohio, https://www.policymattersohio.org/research-policy/sustainable-communities/energy/fracking-in-carroll-county-ohio-an-impact-assessment.

43. Bureau of Labor Market Information, *2017 Annual Ohio Shale Report* (Columbus, OH: Ohio Department of Job and Family Services, 2018), http://ohiolmi.com/OhioShale/2017AnnualShale.pdf.

44. Spencer Hunt and Dan Gearino, "Fracking: So Where's the Economic Boom That Was Promised?," *Columbus Dispatch*, January 28, 2014, https://www.dispatch.com/content/stories/local/2014/01/28/so-wheres-the-boom-that-was-promised.html.

45. Thomas W. Merrill, "Four Questions about Fracking," *Case Western Reserve Law Review* 63, no. 4 (2013): 985.

CHAPTER 7: A PLACE FOR DISASTERS

1. "National Climate Report—Annual 2011," National Oceanic and Atmospheric Administration, accessed August 9, 2019, https://www.ncdc.noaa.gov/sotc/national/201113.

2. "National Climate Report—Annual 2018," National Oceanic and Atmospheric Administration, accessed August 9, 2019, https://www.ncdc.noaa.gov/sotc/national/201813.

3. "The Disaster Declaration Process," Federal Emergency Management Association, last updated January 8, 2018, https://www.fema.gov/disaster-declaration-process.

4. "Disaster Declarations by Year," Federal Emergency Management Association, accessed August 9, 2019, https://www.fema.gov/disasters/year?field_dv2_declaration_type_value=DR.

5. James A. Smith, Mary Lynn Baeck, Alexandros A. Ntelekos, Gabriele Villarini, and Matthias Steiner, "Extreme Rainfall and Flooding from Orographic Thunderstorms in Central Appalachia," *Water Resources Research* 47, no. 4 (April 2011): 1–24, https://doi.org/10.1029/2010WR010190.

6. "National Inventory of Dams," United States Army Corps of Engineers, accessed August 9, 2019, https://nid.sec.usace.army.mil/ords/f?p=105:113:31175734387609.

7. "History of Steel in Johnstown," Johnstown Area Heritage Association, accessed August 11, 2019, https://www.jaha.org/attractions/heritage-discovery-center/johnstown-history/history-steel-johnstown/.

8. David McCullough, *The Johnstown Flood* (New York: Simon and Schuster, 1987).

9. "Facts about the 1889 Flood," Johnstown Area Heritage Association, accessed August 11, 2019, https://www.jaha.org/attractions/johnstown-flood-museum/flood-history/facts-about-the-1889-flood/.

10. Intergovernmental Panel on Climate Change, *Managing the Risks of Extreme Events and Disasters to Advance Climate Change Adaptation* (New York: Cambridge University Press, 2012), 6, https://www.ipcc.ch/report/managing-the-risks-of-extreme-events-and-disasters-to-advance-climate-change-adaptation/.

11. National Research Council, *Advancing the Science of Climate Change* (Washington, DC: National Academies Press, 2010), https://nas-sites.org/americasclimatechoices/sample-page/panel-reports/87-2/.

12. "Climate Monitoring," National Oceanic and Atmospheric Administration, accessed August 11, 2019, https://www.ncdc.noaa.gov/climate-monitoring/.

13. "National Climate Change Viewer," United States Geological Survey, last modified April 26, 2019, https://www2.usgs.gov/landresources/lcs/nccv.asp.

14. U.S. Global Climate Research Program, *Fourth National Climate Assessment*, vol. 2, *Impacts, Risks, and Adaptation in the United States*, pub. online 2018, rev. June 2019, accessed August 11, 2019, https://nca2018.globalchange.gov/.

15. Jennifer Marlon, Peter Howe, Matto Mildenberger, Anthony Leiserowitz, and Xinran Wang, "Yale Climate Opinion Maps 2018," Yale Program on Climate Change Communication, August 7, 2018, https://climatecommunication.yale.edu/visualizations-data/ycom-us-2018.

16. Marlon et al., "Yale Climate Opinion Maps 2018."

17. Kelly Nyks and Jared P. Scott, dirs., *Disruption* (n.p.: PF Pictures, 2014), available at http://watchdisruption.com and https://topdocumentaryfilms.com/disruption/.

18. "Environmental and Climate Justice," National Association for the Advancement of Colored People, accessed August 11, 2019, https://www.naacp.org/programs/entry/climate-justice.

19. Gwen Collman, remarks at the US Department of Health and Human Services 2015 Climate Justice Conference, "Responding to Emerging Health Effects," Research Triangle Park, NC, June 8–9, 2015.

20. U.S. Global Climate Research Program, *Fourth National Climate Assessment*.

21. "Implications of Climate Change," Environmental Protection Agency, Climate Change Adaptation Resource Center (ARC-X), last updated February 18, 2019, https://www.epa.gov/arc-x/implications-climate-change.

22. Kyle Barrett, Patricia Butler, Robert Cooper, Hector Galbraith, Kim Hall, Healy Hamilton, John O'Leary, L. Sneddon, and B. Young, *Understanding Land Use and Climate Change in the Appalachian Landscape, Phase 1: Alternatives for Climate Change Vulnerability*

Assessment: Report to the Appalachian Landscape Conservation Cooperative (Arlington, VA: NatureServe, 2014), https://applcc.org/research/climate-change-vulnerability-group/alternatives-for-climate-change-vulnerability-assessment-report-to-the-appalachian-lcctive.

23. Bertil Forsberg, Lennart Bråbäck, Hans Keune, Mike Kobernus, Martin Krayer von Krauss, Aileen Yang, and Alena Bartonova, "An Expert Assessment on Climate Change and Health—with a European Focus on Lungs and Allergies," *Environmental Health: A Global Access Science Source* 11, supp. 1 (2012): 1–9.

24. Paul T. Leisnham and Steven A. Juliano, "Impacts of Climate, Land Use, and Biological Invasion on the Ecology of Immature *Aedes* Mosquitoes: Implications for La Crosse Emergence," *EcoHealth* 9, no. 2 (June 2012): 217–28, https://doi.org/10.1007/s10393-012-0773-7.

25. Interagency Working Group on Climate Change and Health, *A Human Health Perspective on Climate Change: A Report Outlining the Research Needs on the Human Health Effects of Climate Change* (Research Triangle Park, NC: Environmental Health Perspectives/National Institute of Environmental Health Sciences, 2010), https://www.niehs.nih.gov/health/materials/a_human_health_perspective_on_climate_change_full_report_508.pdf.

26. "Most Recent Asthma Data," Centers for Disease Control and Prevention, last updated March 25, 2019, https://www.cdc.gov/asthma/most_recent_data.htm.

27. Michele Morrone, "Social Determinants of Health Disparities in Appalachia," poster presented at the Minority Health and Health Disparities Grantees' Conference, National Harbor, MD, December 1–3, 2014.

28. Bragg v. Robertson, 54 F. Supp. 2d 635 (S.D. W. Va. 1999), March 3, 1999, https://law.justia.com/cases/federal/district-courts/FSupp2/54/635/2520293/.

29. 64 Fed. Reg. 24 (Feb. 5, 1999), 5778, https://www.gpo.gov/fdsys/pkg/FR-1999-02-05/pdf/99-2825.pdf.

30. Environmental Protection Agency et al., *Mountaintop Mining/Valley Fills in Appalachia: Final Programmatic Environmental Impact Statement*, EPA 9-03-R-05002 (Philadelphia: Environmental Protection Agency, 2005), https://nepis.epa.gov/Exe/ZyPDF.cgi/20005XA6.PDF?Dockey=20005XA6.PDF.

31. "Coal Production Using Mountaintop Removal Mining Decreases by 62% since 2008," Energy Information Administration, July 7, 2015, https://www.eia.gov/todayinenergy/detail.cfm?id=21952.

32. Matthew R. V. Ross, Brian L. McGlynn, and Emily S. Bernhardt, "Deep Impact: Effects of Mountaintop Mining on Surface Topography, Bedrock Structure, and Downstream Waters," *Environmental Science and Technology* 50, no. 4 (2016): 2064–74, https://doi.org/10.1021/acs.est.5b04532.

33. Environmental Protection Agency, *The Effects of Mountaintop Mines and Valley Fills on Aquatic Ecosystems of the Central Appalachian Coalfields*, EPA/600/R-09/138F (Washington, DC: Office of Research and Development, National Center for Environmental Assessment, 2011), https://cfpub.epa.gov/ncea/risk/recordisplay.cfm?deid=225743&CFID=63330774&CFTOKEN=63962894.

34. Laura Kurth, Allan Kolker, Mark Engle, Nicholas Geboy, Michael Hendryx, William Orem, Michael McCawley, Lynn Crosby, Calin Tatu, Matthew Varonka, and Christina DeVera, "Atmospheric Particulate Matter in Proximity to Mountaintop Coal Mines: Sources and Potential Environmental and Human Health Impacts," *Environmental Geochemistry and Health* 37, no. 3 (June 2015): 529–44, https://doi.org/10.1007/s10653-014-9669-5.

35. Travis L. Knuckles, Phoebe A. Stapleton, Valerie C. Minarchick, Laura Esch, Michael McCawley, Michael Hendryx, and Timothy R. Nurkiewicz, "Air Pollution Particulate Matter Collected from an Appalachian Mountaintop Mining Site Induces Microvascular Dysfunction," *Microcirculation* 20, no. 2 (February 2013): 158–69, https://doi.org/10.1111/micc.12014.

36. "Coal Ash (Coal Combustion Residuals, or CCR)," Environmental Protection Agency, last updated July 31, 2019, https://www.epa.gov/coalash.

37. Tennessee Department of Health, *Public Health Assessment: Tennessee Valley Authority (TVA) Kingston Fossil Plant Coal Ash Release* (Nashville: Tennessee Department of Health, 2010), https://www.atsdr.cdc.gov/hac/pha/TVAKingstonFossilPlant/TVAKingstonFossilPlantFinalPHA09072010.pdf.

38. Environmental Protection Agency, "Fact Sheet: Coal Combustion Residuals (CCR): Surface Impoundments with High Hazard Potential Ratings," EPA 530-F-09-006 (June 2009), available via the EPA's National Service Center for Environmental Publications, https://nepis.epa.gov.

39. Marti Maguire, "Duke Energy Pleads Guilty to Environmental Crimes in North Carolina," May 14, 2015, https://www.reuters.com/article/us-duke-energy-spill/duke-energy-pleads-guilty-to-environmental-crimes-in-north-carolina-idUSKBN0NZ25920150514.

40. Reid Frazier, "Leaky Coal Ash Pond Seeks New Pollution Permit from DEP," StateImpact Pennsylvania, National Public Radio, November 29, 2018, https://stateimpact.npr.org/pennsylvania/2018/11/29/leaky-coal-ash-pond-seeks-new-pollution-permit-from-dep/.

Resources

NATIONAL ENVIRONMENTAL HEALTH ORGANIZATIONS

American Public Health Association (APHA): https://apha.org

Member-driven organization of public health professionals; publishes *American Journal of Public Health* and *The Nation's Health;* participates in policy advocacy and educational activities.

National Environmental Health Association (NEHA): https://www.neha.org

Professional organization that sponsors credentials for environmental health professionals, annual education conference, and the *Journal of Environmental Health.*

National Environmental Health Science and Protection Accreditation Council (NEHSPAC): https://www.nehspac.org

Accrediting body for academic environmental health programs.

National Association of County and City Health Officials (NACCHO): https://www.naccho.org

Consists of representatives from local health departments across the country; provides resources, support, and advocacy for public health at the local level.

GOVERNMENTAL ORGANIZATIONS

World Health Organization (WHO): https://www.who.int/phe/en/

International organization dedicated to documenting and improving environmental health across the globe.

Centers for Disease Control and Prevention (CDC), National Center for Environmental Health: https://www.cdc.gov/nceh

Conducts research, surveillance, and educational programs for enhancing environmental health.

National Institute of Environmental Health Sciences (NIEHS): https://www.niehs.nih.gov

Part of the National Institutes of Health (NIH); conducts research, provides grants, and supports policies to promote environmental health.

Healthy People: https://www.healthypeople.gov

Coordinated effort of multiple US agencies to set science-based objectives for improving public health.

ONLINE PUBLICATIONS

Environmental Health Perspectives — http://ehp.niehs.nih.gov

Monthly peer-reviewed journal of research and news published by the National Institute of Environmental Health Sciences.

Environmental Health News — http://www.ehn.org

Independent, foundation-funded news organization that reports, publishes, and contextualizes news stories on environmental topics.

STATE ENVIRONMENTAL AND PUBLIC HEALTH ASSOCIATIONS IN APPALACHIA

Alabama Environmental Health Association: http://www.aeha-online.com
Georgia Environmental Health Association: http://www.geha-online.org
Kentucky Environmental Health Association (formerly Kentucky Association of Milk, Food, and Environmental Sanitarians): http://kyeha.org
Maryland Conference of Local Environmental Health Directors: https://www.mdcounties.org/119/Environmental-Health
North Carolina Public Health Association: https://ncpha.memberclicks.net
Ohio Environmental Health Association: http://www.ohioeha.org
Pennsylvania Association of Milk, Food, and Environmental Sanitarians: https://www.pamfes.org
South Carolina Public Health Association: http://www.scpha.com
Tennessee Public Health Association: https://www.tnpublichealth.org
Virginia Environmental Health Association: http://www.virginiaeha.org
West Virginia Association of Sanitarians: https://wvaos.org/

HEALTH AND ENVIRONMENT AGENCIES IN APPALACHIAN STATES

Alabama

Department of Environmental Management: http://www.adem.state.al.us
Department of Conservation and Natural Resources: https://www.outdooralabama.com
Department of Public Health: http://www.alabamapublichealth.gov

Georgia

Department of Natural Resources: https://www.gadnr.org
Department of Public Health: https://dph.georgia.gov

Kentucky

    Energy and Environment Cabinet
        Environmental Quality Commission: http://eqc.ky.gov
        Department for Natural Resources: https://eec.ky.gov/Natural-Resources
        Department for Environmental Protection: https://eec.ky.gov
          /Environmental-Protection
    Cabinet for Health and Family Services
        Department for Public Health: https://chfs.ky.gov/agencies/dph

Maryland

    Department of the Environment: https://mde.maryland.gov
    Department of Natural Resources: https://dnr.maryland.gov
    Department of Health: https://health.maryland.gov

Mississippi

    Department of Environmental Quality: https://www.mdeq.ms.gov/
    Department of Health: https://msdh.ms.gov/

New York

    Department of Environmental Conservation: http://www.dec.ny.gov
    Department of Health: https://www.health.ny.gov

North Carolina

    Department of Environmental Quality: http://deq.nc.gov
    Division of Public Health: https://publichealth.nc.gov/

Ohio

    Department of Natural Resources: http://ohiodnr.gov/
    Environmental Protection Agency: https://www.epa.state.oh.us/
    Department of Health: https://odh.ohio.gov/

Pennsylvania

    Department of Environmental Protection: https://www.dep.pa.gov
    Department of Conservation and Natural Resources: https://www.dcnr.pa.gov
    Department of Health: https://www.health.pa.gov

South Carolina

    Department of Health and Environmental Control: https://www.scdhec.gov
    Department of Natural Resources: http://www.dnr.sc.gov

Tennessee

    Department of Environment and Conservation: https://www.tn.gov
        /environment
    Department of Health: https://www.tn.gov/health

Virginia

    Department of Environmental Quality: https://www.deq.virginia.gov
    Department of Health: http://www.vdh.virginia.gov

West Virginia

    Department of Environmental Protection: https://dep.wv.gov
    Department of Health and Human Resources: https://dhhr.wv.gov

Suggested Further Reading

Edwards, Grace Toney, JoAnn Aust Asbury, and Ricky L. Cox, eds. *A Handbook to Appalachia: An Introduction to the Region*. Knoxville: University of Tennessee Press, 2006.

Howell, Benita J., ed. *Culture, Environment, and Conservation in the Appalachian South*. Chicago: University of Illinois Press, 2002.

Ludke, Robert L., and Phillip J. Obermiller, eds. *Appalachian Health and Well-Being*. Lexington: University Press of Kentucky, 2012.

Morrone, Michele, and Geoffrey L. Buckley, eds. *Mountains of Injustice: Social and Environmental Justice in Appalachia*. Athens: Ohio University Press, 2011.

Schumann, William, and Rebecca Adkins, eds. *Appalachia Revisited: New Perspectives on Place, Tradition, and Progress*. Lexington: University Press of Kentucky, 2016.

Welch, Wendy, ed. *Public Health in Appalachia: Essays from the Clinic and the Field*. Jefferson, NC: McFarland, 2014.

Index

abandoned mines, 62, 125
acid mine drainage, 62, 125, 137, 146
acid rain, 116
adaptive capacity, 135
ADHS (Appalachian Development Highway
    System), 45–46, 65
AEC (Atomic Energy Commission), 93, 95
AEP. *See* American Electric Power (AEP)
African Americans, 9, 11
Agency for Toxic Substances and Disease
    Registry (ATSDR), 28, 70
Agricultural Marketing Service, 29
agriculture, 53
Agriculture, US Department of (USDA),
    28–29, 81, 89
air: control of pollution, 13, 33, 35, 116; health
    effects, 115–17, 136, 140–41, 143; indoor, 13,
    25, 44, 47; monitoring, 29, 11; outdoor, 23;
    pollution, 3, 17, 24–25, 30, 45, 115–16, 136,
    144; quality, 41, 44, 146, 148; regulations,
    114–15; toxic releases, 99, 102, 105; urban, 7
allergies, 47, 134–35
American Electric Power (AEP), 116–17
American Housing Survey, 64
American Planning Association, 57
American Public Health Association (APHA),
    44, 57
American Reinvestment and Recovery Act, 96
Animal and Plant Health Inspection Service, 29
Appalachian Development Highway System
    (ADHS), 45–46, 65
Appalachian Highlands, 108
Appalachian Mountains, 4, 49, 58, 111
Appalachian Regional Commission (ARC):
    boundaries of the region, 12, 49, 54; cre-
    ation of, 4–6; economic analysis, 8–9, 40,
    65–66; transportation systems, 45
Appalachian Regional Development Act of
    1965, 4, 6
Appalachian Trail, 86

aquifer, 62, 68, 125
ARC. *See* Appalachian Regional Commission
    (ARC)
Arch Coal, 137–38
arsenic, 48, 50, 119
asbestos, 50
asthma, 2, 8, 13, 15, 101; air pollution, 7, 115–16;
    climate change, 132, 134–36, 141; housing,
    47; mining, 139
Athens, OH, 75–78, 90–91
Atomic Energy Commission (AEC), 93, 95
ATSDR (Agency for Toxic Substances and
    Disease Registry), 28, 70

backyard flocks, 86–87
bacteria, 58; water, 63, 73, 109; food, 83, 85–86
Beaver County, PA, 94, 103–5, 115, 141
Bhopal, India, 102
biodiversity, 62
BioWatch, 29
black lung disease, 113
bottom ash, 139
Bud, WV, 59–60, 62, 67–68
Buffalo Creek, 129–30
built environment, 15–16, 23, 29, 35, 39–41, 57;
    and health, 43–44, 46, 56; definition of,
    41; inside environments, 47, 51; outside
    environments, 54–56
Built Environment and Health Initiative, 46
Bush, George H. W., 30
Bush, George W., 138

CAA (Clean Air Act), 69, 115
cancer, 13, 101; climate change and, 135–36; en-
    vironmental cause, 96–97, 146–47; dispar-
    ities, 3, 8, 15; lifestyle causes, 10, 92; lung,
    22, 48–49, 53; mining and, 114; mortality,
    103, 106; pollution and, 103, 106
CAPP (Central Appalachian delivery zone), 111
carbon dioxide, 101, 137, 144

Carroll County, OH, 122–24
CDC (Centers for Disease Control and Prevention), 28; budget, 84; data, 113; disparities, 7, 50–52; estimates of disease, 9, 17; place and health, 44; role in environmental health, 69–70, 85–86, 89; strategies to improve health, 46
census-designated place (CDP), 59
Center for Rural Pennsylvania, 52
Central Appalachian delivery zone (CAPP), 111
CERCLA (Comprehensive Environmental Response, Compensation, and Liability Act), 95
Charleston, WV, 16, 59–60, 68–69, 143
chemicals, 17, 59, 69–70, 116; health effects, 30, 50, 136; fracking, 118–20, 122; organic, 11, 95; mining, 139; regulating, 71; releases, 102, 128; water treatment, 72
Cheshire, OH, 116–17
childhood lead poisoning, 23, 51–52
childhood obesity, 55, 79–80, 89
cholera, 21–22, 25
chronic diseases, 13–14, 20, 27, 82; asthma, 136; connection to pollution, 106, 115, 146; and mining, 110, 112–14; respiratory, 136. *See also* chronic obstructive pulmonary disease (COPD)
city and regional planning, 44
Clean Air Act (CAA), 69, 115
Clean Power Plan, 101
Clean Water Act (CWA), 33, 65, 69, 72; mining, 137–38, 140
Clean Watershed Needs Survey (CWNS), 72
climate change, 23, 30, 130, 137, 146; disasters, 127–28, 130, 141; environmental impacts, 135; food impacts, 85; global impacts, 24–25; health impacts, 134–36, 141; perception, 126, 132, 134; projections, 18, 130–31, 134; vulnerability, 18, 130, 133
climate justice, 132–34
Clinton, Bill, 11
coal, 11, 35; air pollution, 136, 139; camps, 16, 74, 108–10; chemical safety, 70; climate change, 132, 134; company town, 108–10, 114; disasters, 139, 141; economic impacts, 34, 60–61, 101, 110–11, 137; environmental issues, 3, 34, 59–60, 62–63, 125, 146; fatalities, 113–14, 143; health effects, 7, 48–49, 61, 112, 114, 116; history, 107–8, 111, 124, 145; lifecycle, 117; mining, 17; occupational health, 48, 112–13; place-based

public health issues, 114, 117; transporting, 114–15
coal ash, 18, 126, 139–41, 143–45
coal combustion residuals (CCR), 139–40
coal workers' pneumoconiosis (CWP), 113
coalfield, 48–49, 59, 74, 108–9, 112, 137
coal-fired power plant, 101, 115–16
combined sewer overflows (CSOs), 64
Commerce, US Department of, 28
Commissioned Corps, 31
community design, 15–16, 44, 54–56
community gardens, 80
community supported agriculture (CSA), 80
Comprehensive Environmental, Response, Compensation, and Liability Act (CERCLA), 95
construction grants, 65
Consumer Product Safety Commission (CPSC), 30
COPD (chronic obstructive pulmonary disease), 53, 113, 134
cracker plant, 104
credentials, 35
CWP (coal workers' pneumoconiosis), 113

dams, 128, 130
Dan River Spill, 140
DHHS (US Department of Health and Human Services), 28, 31
diabetes, 2, 7–8, 10, 14–15, 19–20, 37, 143; food insecurity, 17, 84, 91; impact, 56, 80
Dimock, PA, 119
disaster declarations, 127–28
disasters, 17, 23, 133, 141; climate change, 18, 130–31; floods, 127–28, 143; human-caused, 3, 18, 127, 136; mining-related, 113, 126, 136–37, 139, 145–46; resilience, 2, 18, 127; response, 29, 31
DOE (US Department of Energy), 93, 95–96
drinking water, 23, 37, 43; access to, 16, 24–25, 108; chemical contamination, 16, 63, 69–70, 95, 140; and fracking, 119–21; infrastructure, 63, 65–66; lead in, 50; microbial contamination, 20, 22, 59–60, 73; radon in, 48–49; regulations, 33, 41, 65; safety, 62, 144; source, 67–68, 71, 97; wells, 95, 120, 126
Duke Energy, 140

Ebola, 24, 28, 84
E. coli, 58, 83, 109

economic(s): climate change, 131, 136; coal, 35, 61–62, 110–11, 117, 137; conditions, 5, 10, 34, 56, 94–96, 103; determinant of health, 2–3, 7, 21, 29, 32, 40, 44, 54, 62; development, 42–43, 45, 57, 65–66, 73, 141; disparities, 6, 8, 17, 57, 99, 145, 147; factor in decisions, 6, 12–14, 36, 53–54, 97–101, 146; food access, 76–77, 82, 84; natural resources, 105, 108, 110–11, 121–25; pollution impact, 99, 101, 105, 116
economic distress, 40, 45, 102, 123
Economic Research Service (ERS), 76
economy-environment debate, 12, 101
education: determinant of health, 29, 143; disparities, 5, 36, 103, 125; environmental health, 29, 35; and health, 2, 9, 24, 37, 48, 55, 57, 106; policy, 56; strategy for health improvement, 38, 54, 74, 84, 90
EIS (Environmental Impact Statement), 137–38
Elk River, 59–60, 63, 68–70, 143
emergency preparedness, 23, 120
emergency response, 33, 128
environmental health, 10, 12, 14, 38, 41–43; accreditation, 35; in Appalachia, 23, 108; climate change, 133; coal, 125, 139, 141, 146; credentials, 35; definition, 18–20; disparities, 15, 72, 90, 133; and the economy, 101–2, 105, 111, 115, 141; and fracking, 118–21; global organizations, 23–26; health departments, 23, 36–37; history, 20–22, 95, 141; inequities, 16, 25, 28, 32, 38, 54, 74, 96–100, 146; national organizations, 28–31; place-based, 50–51, 54, 62; practice, 13, 16, 23, 70, 84; prevention, 27, 85–87, 146; problems in Appalachia, 5–6, 16, 109–10, 114–15, 143; professionals, 18, 27, 35, 67, 74, 83, 132, 143; resources, 128, 146
Environmental Health Specialist, 35
Environmental Impact Assessment (EIA), 46
Environmental Impact Statement (EIS), 137–38
EPA (US Environmental Protection Agency), 30–31, 102; and air quality, 47–49, 115; and climate change, 134; and coal-ash ponds, 140; and coal industry, 34; and fracking, 119–21; history, 95; and mountain-top-removal mining, 137–39; Ohio, 33, 63, 116; and water quality, 60, 67, 69–72
epidemiology, 22–23, 35
ethane cracker plant, 104–5
ethylene, 104–5

farmers' markets, 17, 29, 55, 75, 77, 80–84, 87, 91
FDA (Food and Drug Administration), 28
Federal Emergency Management Agency (FEMA), 29, 127, 140
Federal Mine Safety and Health Review Commission, 30
flood(s), 17, 20, 97, 141, 143; climate change and, 133; disasters, 127–28, 130; health impacts, 65, 128; mountaintop-removal mining, 139
fly ash, 139–40
food: access, 55, 76, 79; economy, 76; inequities, 83. See also food safety; food security; local foods
foodborne illness, 17, 28, 83–85; common causes, 86; outbreaks, 30–31, 87, 144; responding to, 87–88, 90
Food Environment Atlas, 76
Food Environment Index, 76
food safety: environmental health practice, 13, 24, 33–35, 87; farmers' markets, 83; health, 16, 82, 85; inspections, 29, 83; regulatory system, 34, 84; rural areas, 90; schools, 89
Food Safety Inspection Service (FSIS), 29
food security, 2, 84; assistance, 79, 82, 87, 90; children, 79; definition, 76–78; insecurity, 17, 25, 78, 88; local foods, 55, 80, 87; obesity, 55, 79, 82; schools, 89
Forest County, PA, 39–43, 45–46, 53, 57
fracking, 107, 110, 118–25
Freedom Industries, 69

Gallia County, OH, 116
GAO (Government Accountability Office), 119–20
geology, 47–49, 72, 117, 125, 139
Government Accountability Office (GAO), 119–20
Great Stink, 43
greenhouse gas emissions, 25, 34, 131–32
grocery store, 55, 75–76, 78, 81–82, 91
groundwater, 68–69, 95, 98, 141; fracking, 117–18, 120–21, 125

Hancock County, WV, 141
hazardous facilities, 98, 100, 105
hazardous waste, 11, 23, 35, 69; law, 95; management, 13, 33
Health and Human Services, US Department of (DHHS), 28, 31
health departments. See local health departments

health disparities: built environment and, 16, 45, 54; causes of, 28–29, 41, 56–57, 106, 143; climate change and, 133, 141; definition, 6–7; environmental exposures, 146–47; environmental health, 15, 18; equity, comparison with, 9–12, 14; food-related, 90; global, 26, 38; inequities, 23–25, 27, 32; and place, 2, 15–16, 145; resource extraction, 17, 125, 139; rural, 8–9, 57
health education, 24, 37, 55
health equity, 9–10
Health Impact Assessment (HIA), 46, 120
health promotion, 54
healthy communities, 43–44
Healthy Community Design Initiative, 44
Healthy People, 2, 44
healthy places, 43–44, 46
heart disease, 1, 13, 19–20, 53
Homeland Security, US Department of, 28–29, 31
Horsehead Corporation, 104
housing: age of, 52; Forest County, PA, 41; lead, 50–51; radon, 48–49; quality, 3, 44, 47, 64; resources, 5, 123, 146; value, 59
HUD (US Department of Housing and Urban Development), 29, 66

Imboden, VA, 108–10, 114, 117
impoundments, 126, 128, 139–41, 144
indoor air, 13, 25, 44, 47
injustice, environmental, 11–12, 82, 89, 99, 125, 129, 143, 145
Intergovernmental Panel on Climate Change (IPCC), 130
Interior, US Department of, 28
International Sanitary Conference, 21–22

James M. Gavin power plant, 116
Johnstown, PA, 128–30
justice: climate, 132–34; environmental, 11–12, 15, 29, 44, 47, 51, 125; social, 9–10, 82, 108

Kentucky: Appalachian region, 5, 68, 108; climate change, 134; coal, 111, 114–15, 136; flooding, 127, 143; fracking, 118, 122; government, 32, 54; obesity, 80; Paducah, 93; smoking, 53
Kingston Fossil Plant, 126, 140, 143

Labor, US Department of, 28–29
landfills: environmental justice, 11–12, 100; inspections, 6, 36; leachate, 98; siting, 97–98

land-use planning, 15, 24, 46, 55, 57, 99–100, 145
leach field, 73
lead: abatement, 33, 35; blood levels, 50–52; exposure, 16, 44, 53, 145; in gasoline, 13; health effects, 50, 52; paint, 47, 51; poisoning, 23, 51–52; in water, 7, 50
Little Blue Run, 141
local foods: access, 78; economy, 75–77; food safety, 86–88; food security, 55, 80, 87; movement, 55, 80, 90
local health departments, 32, 51, 83; food safety, 84–87; funding, 14, 36; mandates, 23, 33, 37; resources, 35, 52; responsibilities, 65, 121
Logan County, WV, 129
low-income population: climate vulnerability, 133; exposures, 47–48; food access, 76, 78, 81, 90; minority, 9, 11; public health capacity, 23; rural areas, 67, 135; urban areas, 7

malaria, 20, 24
Massey Energy, 113
maximum contaminant levels (MCLs), 69
MCHM (4-Methylclyclohexanemethanol), 69–70
McKibben, Bill, 132
median household income (MHI), 42, 59
Medicaid, 34, 51
mental health, 2, 40, 45
mercury, 50
microbes, 69, 73, 85
Mine Safety and Health Administration (MSHA), 62, 112
Montcoal, WV, 113
mosquitoes, 13–14, 20–21, 23–24, 36, 47, 135
mountaintop-removal mining (MTR), 136; environmental consequences, 3, 10, 111, 137–39; health effects, 114; pollutants, 136; technique, 137

National Academy of Medicine, 130
National Academy of Sciences, 130
national ambient air quality standards (NAAQS), 115
National Association for the Advancement of Colored People (NAACP), 133
National Center for Environmental Health, 28, 69
National Climate Assessment, 132, 134
National Environmental Health Science and Protection Accreditation Council (EHAC), 35

National Health and Nutrition Examination Survey (NHANES), 50, 79
National Institute of Environmental Health Sciences (NIEHS), 28–29, 70, 133–35
National Institute of Occupational Safety and Health (NIOSH), 112
National Institutes of Health (NIH), 28, 70
National Inventory of Dams, 128
National Oceanic Atmospheric Administration (NOAA), 127, 131
National Radon Action Plan, 48
National Research Council, 130
National School Lunch Act, 88
National Science Foundation (NSF), 30
National Small Flows Clearing House, 109
National Toxicology Program (NTP), 69
natural gas: activism, 63; economic impact, 101, 105, 111, 117–18, 122; energy impact, 35, 94, 104, 107; environmental impacts, 62, 141; health impacts, 119, 125; history, 3, 12, 17; regulation, 33
NHANES (National Health and Nutrition Examination Survey), 50, 79
NIEHS (National Institute of Environmental Health Sciences), 28–29, 70, 133–35
nitrogen dioxide, 115–16, 144
NOAA (National Oceanic Atmospheric Administration), 127, 131
norovirus, 83, 85–86
North Carolina: climate change, 134; farmers' markets, 81; floods, 127; food, 87; and smoking, 53; Warren County, 11
nuclear energy, 93–96, 104–5
Nuclear Regulatory Commission (NRC), 30, 95

Oak Ridge, TN, 93
obesity: and diabetes, 56, 84; environmental causes, 13–16, 44, 55–56; food access, 79, 82; public health, 37; rates, 2, 16–17, 40, 79–80
occupational safety, 23, 29, 35, 112
Occupational Safety and Health Act, 112
Occupational Safety and Health Administration (OSHA), 30, 112
Ohio Environmental Protection Agency (Ohio EPA), 33, 63, 116
OSHA (Occupational Safety and Health Administration), 30, 112
outdoor air quality, 23
overburden, 137–38
ozone, 116, 135–36

Paducah, KY, 93
Pan American Health Organization (PAHO), 24–25
Pan American Sanitary Code, 25
Paris, KY, 115
particulate matter (PM), 116, 136
Pavillion, WY, 119
PCBs, 11, 95
Pennsylvania, 32; Beaver County, 94, 103–5; climate change, 134; coal, 34, 114–15, 141; floods, 127; fracking, 118–19, 122; health departments, 42; lead exposure, 51–52; rural, 7, 39; Shippingport, 141; water quality, 65, 68
Performance Coal, 113
physical activity, 44–45, 55–57, 61
physiographic region, 107
Pike County, OH, 93–94, 96–97, 99, 103, 105
place, concept of, 4
place-based disparities, 7, 145
place-based exposures, 10, 22, 25, 38, 50
place-based inequities, 12, 26
place-based solutions, 13–15, 23, 28
plague, 21
Plan4Health, 57
polio, 24
pollution havens, 98–100, 102–5; hypothesis, 98
Portsmouth Gaseous Diffusion Plant (PORTS), 93, 105
poverty, 5, 45, 94, 143; ARC analysis, 8; built environment, 47–51; climate change, 135; coal, 34; and environment, 27, 61; food, 75–77, 88–89; and health, 2, 10, 36, 80; health inequites, 9, 25; and pollution, 103; rural, 87; vulnerability, 7; War on Poverty, 6
Poverty-Environment Initiative (PEI), 26–27
power plant: coal, 49, 101, 114–16, 141; nuclear, 30, 94, 104–5; siting, 98–100
public health, 2, 27; agencies, 14, 28–30, 32–33, 71; capacity, 141, 143, 145; and climate change, 131–36; definition of, 12–13, 18; and economy, 2, 5–6, 8, 10, 17, 95; funding, 23, 34, 52, 64, 66, 84, 87, 90; history, 20–22, 71; local, 36–37, 65, 68, 146; and place, 7, 38, 49, 54–55, 62, 80, 126; and planning, 43–46, 56–57, 100; professionals, 12, 35, 54; regulations, 27–28, 67; researchers, 79; success story, 51, 110
Public Health Assessment, 140

publicly owned treatment works (POTWs), 33, 64
public water system, 42, 62, 64, 67–68

quality of life, 2, 66, 114, 136

race, 7, 9, 11, 20, 29, 99
radiation, 23, 47–48, 72, 96, 136
radon, 16, 47–50, 53–54, 145
recession, 61, 122
Registered Environmental Health Specialist (REHS), 35
Registered Sanitarian (RS), 35
Research Triangle Environmental Health Collaborative, 120
resilience, 127
Rio Political Declaration on Social Determinants of Health, 25
Robert Wood Johnson Foundation (RWJF), 3, 9, 40, 61, 76
rural places: challenges, 64; definition of, 52; economy, 110, 135, 147; environmental conditions, 16, 49, 51; environmental justice, 11–12, 133, 143; food access, 76, 78–84, 90; health disparities, 7, 16, 25, 57; physical activity, 56; place, 45, 55; planning, 46; pollution, 115; resources for public health, 6, 14, 38, 42, 74, 146; siting hazardous facilities, 93–94, 97, 99, 125; vs. urban, 25, 60, 87, 134; water infrastructure, 66–68, 72–73

Safe Drinking Water Act, 33, 67
Salmonella, 83, 85–87
Salt Fork Hunting & Fishing Club, 129
sanitary reform movement, 43
sanitation, 13, 21–22, 24–25, 31, 47
school lunch, 88–90
School Nutrition Association (SNA), 89
SCI Forest, 40, 42
secondhand smoke, 16, 47, 53, 145
selective catalytic reduction (SCR), 116
septic system, 33, 41, 63–65, 68, 73, 109
sewers, 41–42, 63–66, 72
shale gas, 17, 110, 120, 122, 124, 141
Shell Chemical, 104
Shippingport, PA, 94, 104–5, 141
smoking: bans, 54, 144; behavior, 10, 18, 40, 61, 143; cessation, 22, 37; rates, 48, 53
SNAP (Supplemental Nutrition Assistance Program), 37, 78–79, 81

social determinants of health, 2, 24, 26, 29, 38, 145
social justice, 9–10, 82
State Revolving Loan Fund, 65
steel industry, 129
storms, 127
stroke, 135
suburb, 6, 9, 44, 54, 81
sulfur, 116
sulfur dioxide, 114–15, 144
sulfuric acid, 62, 116
surgeon general, 31, 35
sustainability, 26, 44, 11, 124–25

Tennessee Valley Authority (TVA), 30, 109
Third World, 26
Three Mile Island, 94
tobacco, 44, 53–54
Toxic Release Inventory (TRI), 102, 116
Toxic Substances Control Act (TSCA), 70
trains, 62, 108, 114–15
transportation, 6, 37, 43–46, 56–57, 145
Transportation, US Department of, 28
TVA (Tennessee Valley Authority), 30, 109

US Army Corps of Engineers (USACE), 137–38
US Census, 41, 51, 59, 88
US Coast Guard, 29
US Congress: authority, 31, 119, 134; budget, 65, 70, 96; House of Representatives, 34, 70, 89; laws, 4, 50, 88, 95, 112; public health, 34, 36
USDA (US Department of Agriculture), 28–29, 81, 89
US Department of Energy (DOE), 93, 95–96
US Energy Information Administration (EIA), 105, 111
US Environmental Protection Agency (EPA), 30–31, 102
US Geological Survey (USGS), 131–32
US Public Health Service (USPHS), 31, 44
unemployment, 29, 34, 61, 96, 103, 143; impact on health programs, 36; and job promises, 100, 111, 124; and poverty, 5, 40, 45, 94
unfunded mandates, 34, 70
United Church of Christ, 11
United Nations Climate Summit, 133
United Nations Environment Program (UNEP), 24, 26
Upper Big Branch Mine, 113–14
uranium enrichment, 93–96, 144

Village of Euclid, 100
Virginia, 108–9
viruses, 85–86
vulnerability, 130, 134–35

Walmart, 77, 80, 108
War on Coal, 34, 101, 139
War on Poverty, 6
Warren County, NC, 11–12
wastewater, 23, 41; coal mining impacts, 125, 130; and economic development, 66; infrastructure, 33, 42, 63–65, 72, 108; onsite, 37, 64–65; sanitation, 13, 25, 72–73; treatment, 16, 71, 109; untreated, 25, 63–64, 71, 74
Watauga County, NC, 87
water quality, 6, 17, 41; coal mining impacts on, 110; environmental impacts on, 46, 62–64; fracking impacts on, 121; laws, 33

weather, 116; extreme events, 127–28, 132–33, 135, 146; related disasters, 17–18, 133; related health impacts, 135, 141
wells: drinking water, 33, 65, 67, 73, 95, 120–21, 126, 140; injection, 102; monitoring, 98, 119; natural gas, 17, 118, 122, 124, 146
WHO (World Health Organization), 22, 24
Wise County, WV, 108, 110
World Conference on Social Determinants of Health, 24
World Health Assembly, 24
World Health Organization (WHO), 22, 24
Wyoming County, WV, 58–61, 74

yellow fever, 21, 25

Zika virus, 24, 28
zoning, 99–100

Printed by Printforce, United Kingdom